SCALING UP HEALTH INNOVATIONS IN AFRICA

Prospects and Challenges

Health practitioners have successfully developed evidence-based health innovations to solve public health problems. However, challenges remain in translating and scaling up these innovations to save and improve lives in Africa. *Scaling Up Health Innovations in Africa* focuses on the lessons learned from scaling up health innovations across the continent.

Obidimma Ezezika provides engaging and insightful evidence on the challenges and triumphs of taking health innovations to scale, drawing from hundreds of interviews with practitioners on the ground. The book includes stories, anecdotes, and lessons from experiences in eleven African countries, including Kenya, Rwanda, Tanzania, Nigeria, Burkina Faso, Uganda, and Mozambique. It addresses the unique socio-cultural, financial, and logistical constraints faced in these regions, alongside insights, successes, and next steps for scaling innovations within the African context.

The book critically emphasizes the importance of understanding how implementation science can aid in scaling up innovations in Africa. While there have been disparate works on scaling specific health innovations in Africa, a unified series of cases is needed from an implementation science perspective to create generalizable lessons and principles. Ultimately, *Scaling Up Health Innovations in Africa* offers valuable insights around implementation strategies that translate health innovations to achieve broad impact.

OBIDIMMA EZEZIKA is an associate professor in the Faculty of Health Sciences and the director of the Global Health and Innovation Lab at Western University.

Scaling Up Health Innovations in Africa

Prospects and Challenges

OBIDIMMA EZEZIKA

UNIVERSITY OF TORONTO PRESS
Toronto Buffalo London

Toronto Buffalo London
utppublishing.com
Printed in the USA

ISBN 978-1-4875-5012-7 (cloth)
ISBN 978-1-4875-5225-1 (paper)
ISBN 978-1-4875-5379-1 (EPUB)
ISBN 978-1-4875-5295-4 (PDF)

Library and Archives Canada Cataloguing in Publication

Title: Scaling up health innovations in Africa : prospects and challenges / Obidimma Ezezika.
Names: Ezezika, Obidimma, 1979– author
Description: Includes bibliographical references and index.
Identifiers: Canadiana (print) 2025014980X | Canadiana (ebook) 20250149834 | ISBN 9781487550127 (cloth) | ISBN 9781487552251 (paper) | ISBN 9781487552954 (PDF) | ISBN 9781487553791 (EPUB) | ISBN 9781487560874 (OA)
Subjects: LCSH: Medical care—Africa. | LCSH: Medical policy—Africa. | LCSH: Medical innovations—Africa. | LCSH: Public health—Africa.
Classification: LCC RA545 .E94 2025 | DDC 362.1096—dc23

Cover design: Kristjan Buckingham
Cover image: iStock.com/MicroStockHub

We wish to acknowledge the land on which the University of Toronto Press operates. This land is the traditional territory of the Wendat, the Anishnaabeg, the Haudenosaunee, the Métis, and the Mississaugas of the Credit First Nation.

University of Toronto Press acknowledges the financial support from the University of Toronto Libraries in making the open access version of this title available.

University of Toronto Press acknowledges the financial support of the Government of Canada, the Canada Council for the Arts, and the Ontario Arts Council, an agency of the Government of Ontario, for its publishing activities.

Canada Council for the Arts | Conseil des Arts du Canada

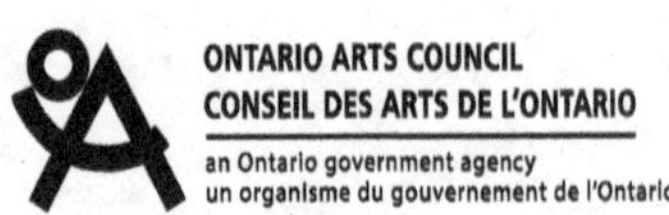

Funded by the Government of Canada | Financé par le gouvernement du Canada

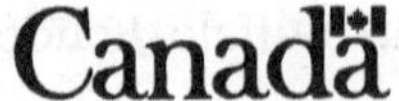

Contents

Acknowledgments

This book is the result of the generous contributions, sharp insights, and tireless support of many individuals, each of whom played a vital role in its development.

I am especially grateful to **Kishif Fatima**, whose extensive editing, careful proofreading, and thoughtful comments across multiple drafts brought clarity and depth to the manuscript. **Omolola Olorunbiyi** provided detailed feedback and proofreading across several chapters, helping to refine and sharpen the book's key messages. **Jenny Gong** was instrumental in the early stages, contributing to the conceptualization of the book and enriching initial discussions with fresh ideas and critical insight.

The development of Chapter 1 was shaped by the expert support of **Kathryn Barrett** whose library and data expertise laid a solid foundation, and by **Suleyman Demi**, who provided thoughtful feedback on early drafts of this pivotal chapter. **Jennifer Heng** offered invaluable feedback on the polio chapter, while **Meron Mengistu** contributed thoughtful and detailed feedback on Chapter 11, focused on the HPV vaccine. **Edward Ameyaw** shared insightful feedback on Chapter 7, which explores mHealth, and **Selina Quibrantar** provided helpful suggestions on early drafts of Chapter 6, *Vitamin A Has a Story to Tell.*

I would also like to thank **Bethlehem Tesfaye** for her careful proofreading, and **Thuvaraha Jeyakumaran** and **Raza Haider** for their diligent research support throughout several chapters of the book.

Special thanks go to the outstanding editorial team at University of Toronto Press. **Jodi Litvin**, our acquisitions editor, championed this project from the outset and guided it with confidence and care. **Ryan Pidhayny**, managing editor for *Scaling Up Health Innovations in Africa,* ensured a seamless production process, and **Dawn Hunter**, our meticulous copy editor, brought precision and polish to the final text.

Finally, I wish to express my heartfelt appreciation to the **past and present members of the Global Health & Innovation Lab** and the **African Centre for Innovation & Leadership Development**, whose energy, creativity, and commitment to equitable health solutions have continuously inspired this work. Though too numerous to name individually, your collective contributions—through research, discussion, design, and collaboration—are deeply woven into the spirit and substance of this book.

To each of you, thank you for your care, generosity, and commitment. Your support echoes throughout every chapter.

SCALING UP HEALTH INNOVATIONS IN AFRICA

1

They Came, They Saw, They Scaled: Health Innovations for Impact

The objective may be global, but implementation is always local. The strategy for smallpox eradication did not change from country to country, but the local culture determined which tactics were most useful. Only the specific locality can provide information on who is sick, who is hiding from the vaccinators, when people are available for vaccination, how to hire watch guards, or how to secure the cooperation of the community. In all cultures, an approach of respect for local customs is needed.

– William Herbert Foege, Former Director,
Centers for Disease Control and Prevention

Fourteen years ago, I interviewed Ananda Chakrabarty, a microbiologist who was the first to create and patent a genetically engineered microbe to break crude oil down into water and carbon dioxide – with massive potential for cleaning up oil spills.[1]

As an early career microbiologist, I was eager to learn the secrets of this scientific breakthrough and the steps that followed for it to have a real-world impact. But other than being awarded a patent, that microbe was literally sitting on the shelf. The history of innovation is littered with failure. But to see the potential success of this one trapped in the lab was shocking to my younger and more idealistic self.

Over the years, I came to realize how often the bridge from the lab to the village breaks. Every scientist, engineer, politician, and entrepreneur experiences the *delivery gap* at one time or another. Knowing what works is no guarantee it will reach the people it's intended for.

Maybe Africa knows this story best of all, particularly in global health. For example, over 400,000 children died of diarrhea in 2021, making it one of the world's leading causes of child mortality. Why is it that oral rehydration solutions, which cost just pennies and reduce deaths from childhood diarrhea by over 90%, reach only 4 in 10 children? This situation mirrors that of numerous health innovations in Africa.

According to the World Health Organization (WHO), health innovations refer to the development of effective, accessible, and improved policies, systems, services, and products focused on improving the target population's health.[2] It is vital that such innovations are based on scientific evidence that demonstrates each innovation's effectiveness and integrates the expertise of diverse professionals, such as clinicians and specialists, holistic values and expectations from the target population, and key research findings.[3] The implementation of such innovations has to improve the delivery and accessibility of healthcare. For example, after years of research indicating the convenience and accessibility of digital health technologies, such as smartphone applications and text-messaging programs, they have become an integral part of cardiovascular healthcare.[4] MomConnect, a national health innovation tool launched in South Africa to connect mothers to prenatal and postnatal care, was scaled to the point that over 1.7 million pregnant women in 95% of the nation's public health facilities were receiving health information messages from the program,[5] which I discuss in Chapter 7.

Despite the examples of successful implementations of evidence-based health innovations, there are barriers to successful implementation and sustainability in Africa. The lack of resources, including personnel and infrastructure (e.g., unreliable power, limited operational equipment), inadequate policies, difficulty in community integration with technology, poor understanding about scaling up, and finances pose barriers to the successful implementation of such innovations, specifically in middle- and low-income countries.[6,7]

A case study in Ghana identified that despite the nation's vision for implementing evidence-based innovations, existing policies, funding allocations for research, and the healthcare sector pose barriers.[8] Similar trends have been observed in Uganda, where the lack of policies, funding allocation, and effective coordination among key partners require refinement to support the implementation of such innovations).[9] Therefore, such barriers must be addressed to ensure evidence-based health innovations are scaled up.

Scaling up refers to building and strengthening infrastructures, such as health systems and organizations, to support and sustain full-scale implementation of practice. The WHO[10] defined scaling up as an effort to increase the impact of health innovation to benefit more people while fostering sustainable development of policies. The WHO recognizes that scaling up involves various elements, including the innovation, the innovation team, the users, and the environment (i.e., policies, health sector, bureaucracy) in which the scaling up takes place. Scaling up aims to build sustainability around implementations by adapting to the needs of local communities, engaging key interested groups, and increasing the spread of innovations. For example, post-abortion care (PAC) was introduced to many public health systems in 1994.[11]

In Bolivia and Mexico, the focus of PAC was to provide clinical treatment to women who had complications from abortions while also providing them with counselling on contraceptives. However, the numbers of unsafe abortions are increasing and continue to raise concern. Researchers recognized PAC as a secondary prevention strategy; therefore, scaling-up strategies were implemented in hopes of improving advocacy, health system capacities, and access to technologies and equipment. After developing a conceptual framework, increasing funding of and resources for the program, and ensuring continual monitoring and research of existing PAC procedures, the program was scaled up. The current program now has increased political commitment to PAC and has improved access to equipment and other resources dedicated to PAC, demonstrating the clear connection between scaling up and sustainable innovations.[11]

In this chapter, I explain why it is crucial to focus implementation research in the African context. Africa reached a population of 2.5 billion by 2025; however, the continent still has high numbers of morbidities and mortalities. Most of these morbidities and mortalities are preventable through the scaling up of innovations and interventions. Thus, this is an urgent issue that needs our attention. Africa presents unique constraints and challenges to scaling interventions; the best way to learn is through examining case studies and how implementation challenges were overcome in different scenarios. The eradication of smallpox in Africa is a fitting example.

The excerpt at the beginning of this chapter from the book *House on Fire: The Fight to Eradicate Smallpox* by William Herbert Foege[12] highlights the importance of aligning global initiatives with local contexts for effective, locally informed solutions to global problems. While smallpox eradication was a universal goal, its success depended on how well the strategy adapted to local practices, beliefs, challenges, and opportunities. This underscores that not only is respecting and integrating local knowledge and customs a matter of cultural sensitivity, but it is also necessary for a practical approach to achieving public health goals. Even though the strategy for smallpox eradication did not change from country to country, the local culture determined which strategies were useful and which were not; using smallpox and other cases such as HIV, malaria, and COVID-19, I demonstrate how implementation science has been used in Africa and discuss the prospects and constraints of institutions scaling up implementation science in the region.

Role of Implementation Science in Scaling Up

Implementation science aims to promote evidence-based practice to improve and provide effective solutions to current health concerns. However, there can be a disconnect between research and practice without adequate resources, infrastructural support, and real-world applicability. For over a decade, implementation science has expanded to bridge the gap between health research and real-life application. In the research process, there is a shift from dissemination science (uptake of an intervention) to implementation science (real-world application) that remains difficult to distinguish. Consequently, describing the process of implementation science remains a challenge.

Curran[13] used a teaching tool to help individuals think like implementation scientists, outlining five points: describing the intervention (describing the thing), using effectiveness research (analyzing whether the thing works), conducting implementation research (understanding how to do the thing), applying implementation strategies (determining what we do to help do the thing), and analyzing implementation outcomes (establishing how much and how well the thing is done). The aim is to provide clarity and highlight the importance of this research tool. I consider this one of the simplest definitions of implementation science.

An example of the definition in the context of oral rehydration solution (ORS), used for the treatment of dehydration caused by diarrhea, is apropos. ORS can be regarded as the "thing." In fact, studies have suggested that if every child who needs ORS gets it, 93% of child deaths caused by diarrhea could be prevented.[14] Since its first use in the 1960s, ORS has saved more than 70 million lives, and since 1978, the WHO has implemented ORS use in many countries to treat diarrhea.[15] In communities in which ORS was promoted, mortality resulting from diarrhea decreased by 69%, compared with communities that did not receive the promotion.[14] Moreover, with advancements in oral rehydration therapy (ORT) interventions, like polymer-based ORS, individuals suffering from diarrhea have experienced reduced amounts of stool expulsion 24 hours after treatment and about an 8-hour shorter duration of diarrhea.[16] Implementation research analyzes ORS through a local context, specific to a country, to understand the gaps and learn from previous uptake of ORS (understanding how to do the thing). Implementation strategies used include increasing accessibility/availability, addressing opposing beliefs regarding ORS treatment, engaging key partners, creating incentives, and ensuring the intervention design is applicable to that specific community (determining what we do to help do the thing). Implementation outcomes depend on many factors, including the local applicability, because in some communities, ORS may be more challenging to implement (establishing how much and how well the thing is done). So, we see that shifting from uptake (dissemination) of an intervention to a wide-scale global health approach (implementation) requires knowledge of both the purpose and the process of implementation science.

Implementation science is essentially the promotion of evidence-based standardized practice that focuses on the systematic uptake of research findings to improve and advance current methods.[17] One of the greatest challenges in science is effectively transferring the results that are found in research to real-world situations. Therefore, a multitude of implementation science frameworks have emerged with six focus areas: adaptability, capacity-building strategies, assessment strategies, planning, support strategies, and future application improvement.[18] For example, the active implementation framework uses a multi-level approach. First, one identifies the intervention and then assesses previous trials of the intervention for required resources, before the initial implementation.[19]

In many cases, implementation science becomes vital in scaling up health innovations in Africa. I provide four examples. The first is in Ghana, where high fertility rates paired with social and economic consequences (i.e., poverty) was discovered to be a consequence of reduced contraceptive use. More than 70% of Ghanaians lived more than eight kilometres away from the nearest healthcare facilities and providers in 1990.[20] Given these challenges, a pilot project called the Community-Based Health Planning and Services (CHPS) was launched in Navrongo, in the Upper East Region of Ghana. This program aimed to promote the use of contraceptives, make healthcare more accessible, and address the underlying concerns that inhibited quality healthcare delivery in Ghana. As part of monitoring and evaluation measures, focus group interviews were conducted with community members, healthcare staff, and district leaders throughout the project to assess the impact of the project, community engagement, and service strategies. In its initial phase, facilities were built to increase accessibility to healthcare.

Two years after project implementation, the implementers sought to bring healthcare to more communities by deploying nurses to remote communities. Soon after, the Navrongo pilot project was deemed a success as childhood mortality and fertility rates declined.[20] In 1999, the program expanded across Ghana. The program aimed to replicate an approach in Bangladesh while tailoring the program to the needs of remote and rural communities in Ghana. District management health teams expanded their efforts to provide door-step healthcare across Ghana, with services such as immunizations, family planning, health education, treatment of minor illnesses, and more. In 2020, out of 6445 demarcated CHPS zones, 5987 were functional, allowing CHPS to contribute heavily to service delivery and bridge the gap between access and service delivery.[21] In 2015, CHPS contributed 8.1% to outpatient department attendance and continues to provide 54.7% of postnatal care services, 33% of family planning services, and 51% of expanded immunization programs.[21]

A second example is a case study in South Africa on improving prevention of mother-to-child transmission (PMTCT) of HIV. The PMTCT of HIV is a priority in South Africa, given that more than 20% of pregnant women in South Africa are infected with HIV.[22] The PMTCT program is a multi-step approach to care for mothers and children and to prevent transmission. The program was implemented in 2000 and aimed to test pregnant mothers for HIV, initiate antiretroviral treatment, and test infants for infection six weeks after birth.[23, 25] This program was initially implemented in three districts in which the effectiveness and applicability of the program were assessed.

The Department of Health then supported the scaling of this initiative, with efforts focused on quality improvement as they collaborated with five more districts across South Africa and recognized the gaps in service delivery at the reproductive, maternal, postnatal, and child health stages.[24] In 2010, local partners and district health teams conducted bottleneck analyses at each stage of the PMTCT program to assess the obstacles in service delivery. Using their findings, they developed an individualized framework to improve the accessibility and efficiency of the PMTCT program by scaling it up. They identified seven indicators, from the number of pregnant women presenting for their first antenatal visit and gestational age at first visit to the number of HIV-exposed infants who were tested for HIV and those found to be HIV positive.[25] In 2012, the analyses were repeated across districts to assess the effectiveness of the framework. As part of the scaling-up initiative, a monitoring system was also developed to notify healthcare teams of critical points of the PMTCT program. As the program expanded across the country, health teams continued to monitor discrepancies in service delivery and quality of care. The continual effort to implement key findings to improve the quality of the program has led to the program being fully scaled up across the country in all 52 districts, with visible improvements in PMTCT of HIV. As a result of the PMTCT guidelines in South Africa, the incidence of paediatric HIV infections declined by 84% between 2009 and 2015.[25]

Third is a case study of the rapid scale up of antiretroviral therapy (ART) for HIV patients in Rwanda, a country in East Africa. In 1983, the first case of HIV was reported in Rwanda. By 1986, the country conducted its first population-based seroprevalence survey and reported an urban prevalence of 18% and a rural prevalence of 1%.[26] The efforts to curb the spread of HIV in the country were disrupted by the 1994 genocide.[27] Rape was used as a weapon of war against over 250,000 women, driving a dramatic surge in HIV infections.[28] To combat the AIDS epidemic, Rwanda re-established the National Programme for HIV/AIDS Control (PNLS) in 1995.[27] The initial objective of the PNLS was to educate Rwandans about HIV prevention and treatment. However, the high cost of HIV treatment was a significant challenge. In 1999, treatment costs were as high as USD 6065 per patient per year, with antiretroviral prices accounting for 92% of the overall cost of care. Only 202 Rwandans who were HIV positive at the time could afford the medication.[29]

To scale up HIV treatment, the Universal Treatment Program was launched in 2000, initially funded by the government, to provide ART at the Kigali Teaching Hospital.[27] In 2002, Rwanda received USD 30.5 million from the World Bank to increase access to HIV testing, social impact mitigation, and ART purchases for those in need. In the same year, the US President's Emergency Plan for AIDS Relief was initiated, and Rwanda was awarded USD 39 million to support increased access to ART and PMTCT.[27] To further increase access to antiretroviral drugs for the poor populations, Rwanda leveraged the World Trade Organization amendment to the Trade-Related Aspects of Intellectual Property agreement by awarding a contract to the Canadian generic manufacturer Apotex to produce the triple combination AIDS drug Apo-TriAvir on its behalf in 2008. By September 2008, the first shipment of 6.8 million pills arrived in Rwanda.[30]

Rwanda's rapid expansion of ART is a remarkable success story. Before 2002, fewer than 100 Rwandans had received ART; however, by 2015, this number had risen to over 150,000.[27] Furthermore, the country reached universal coverage of ART at a CD4 cell count of 200 cells/mm^3 in 2007 and raised the threshold for initiating ART to 350 cells/mm^3 in 2008.

A fourth example is the Malawi Chipatala Cha Pa Foni (CCPF) project. Malawi was known to have the highest maternal, newborn, and child mortality rates in the world, with a maternal mortality ratio of

675 maternal deaths per 1 million live births and an under-five mortality rate of 112 deaths per 1000 births.[31] In response to these issues, the Malawi Ministry of Health partnered with Village Reach (a non-profit organization) to adopt the CCPF in 2013 as a tool to improve maternal, newborn, and child health (MNCH).[32] The CCPF (meaning "Health Centre by Phone") is a service with a hotline, voice and text-based tips, and reminders that provides medical guidance and referrals on reproductive and MNCH to women and guardians of young children in rural areas without other access to health information.[32]

Initially, the CCPF was implemented in a single district in 2011. In 2013, with the partnership of the Ministry of Health, CCPF was implemented in 4 (Balaka, Nkhotakota, Mchinji, and Mulanje) of the 28 districts in Malawi. These districts were chosen based on reports of high mortality rates and the considerable travel time needed to reach a medical facility.[31,32] Following a positive impact evaluation of the program in 2013,[31] CCPF's implementation expanded to nine districts (Balaka, Ntcheu, Mchinji, Nkhotakota, Mulanje, Machinga, Dedza, Salima, and Zomba) in 2017. Also, the Ministry of Health institutionalized the initiative within the public health system to serve Malawians in all 28 districts.[33] Although the initial goal of CCPF was on MNCH and providing advice for appropriate healthcare-seeking behaviour, its mission has expanded. The CCPF now includes many relevant health topics, such as nutrition, infectious disease, water, sanitation, and hygiene, following recommendations from Malawi's Ministry of Health.[34] Youth services were introduced, increasing access to sexual and reproductive health information for young people.[34]

Reaching Grand Convergence

As defined by the Lancet Commission on Investing in Health, *grand convergence* is the reduction of preventable infections and child and maternal mortality to universally low levels.[35] This can be achieved by scaling up evidence-based innovations and technological advancement, which has had significant implications for the health of populations in high-income countries. The advancements have helped to enhance labour and delivery, child health, and maternal health tools that have evidently decreased maternal mortality, infant mortality, and infectious disease mortality in high-income populations.[36] Unfortunately, low- and middle-income countries (LMICs) have not experienced the same technological advancements and remain impacted by high morbidity and mortality rates. This has created a divergence (separation) between high-income countries' and LMICs' morbidity/mortality rates. However, Rwanda experienced the most significant reduction in child mortality in recorded history. Suppose other LMICs could replicate the decline in child mortality, along with an increase in domestic health investment and a realignment of donor priorities. In that case, most countries could reach grand convergence by 2035.[35]

Similarly, suppose there were a significant convergence of crucial health outcomes between LMICs and high-income countries. In that case, grand convergence can be achieved by 2030.[36] This grand convergence would be evident through reduced infection and maternal and infant mortality rates. To date, high-income countries like Sweden and some LMICs like China have experienced grand convergence.[36] There is evidence that the scaling up of various health innovations and technologies in LMICs, like Africa, could have major implications for population health. To reach grand convergence, scaling up of a wide range of interventions and innovations is required. It is essential to highlight that substantial investment is needed to scale up initiatives for LMICs.[36] For example, Africa has the highest maternal mortality rate in the world.[37] Postpartum hemorrhage is a leading cause of maternal death worldwide.[38] In 2012, the WHO recommended uterine balloon tamponade (UBT) for treating postpartum hemorrhage.[39] According to Herrick et al.'s[40] model study, widespread use of UBTs in clinics and hospitals in sub-Saharan Africa can save 6547 lives (an 11% reduction in maternal deaths), avert 10,823 surgeries, and prevent 634 cases of severe anemia each year. However, because of the high cost of the devices, which range from USD 125 to USD 350 for a one-time use, UBT is still widely underused and inaccessible in LMICs.[40]

African countries can reach grand convergence by investing considerably in the health sector. According to Jamison et al.,[41] for low-income countries to achieve grand convergence by 2035, it will cost an additional USD 23 billion per year from 2016 to 2025 and USD 27 billion per year from 2026 to 2035. For lower-middle-income countries, it will cost an additional USD 38 billion per year from 2016 to 2025, and USD 53 billion per year from 2026 to 2035.[41] Increased investment in developing new health tools is required. Policy and implementation research to guide the scale-up of new and existing tools is also necessary.

Grand convergence in Africa is possible if the huge "delivery gap" can be closed.[42] The delivery gap is the difference between what is known to be effective and what is delivered. Scaling up the coverage of existing health interventions like immunization, vaccination, and ORT in Africa could decrease maternal, neonatal, and child deaths by 85%.[43] However, this requires that health disparities within African countries be addressed.[44] Everyone in the country, regardless of socio-economic status, must have access to high-quality healthcare services.

To achieve convergence, most LMICs would require an under-five mortality rate of 16 per 1000 live births, an annual AIDS death rate of 8 per 100,000 population, and an annual tuberculosis death rate of 4 per 100,000 population, according to Global Health 2035.[41] Abraham Horwitz, the first Latin American director of the Pan American Sanitary Bureau, characterized Chile, Costa Rica, and Cuba as a trio of what he called "countries that cope."[45] Despite political alteration, economic crisis, and epidemic outbreaks, these countries overcame these hurdles to dramatically reduce infectious and child mortality rates through the scaling up of healthcare interventions.[45]

As of 2011, the annual child mortality rate in the aforementioned countries was less than 12 per 1000 live births.[46] Rwanda, with a population of about 13.5 million people, has also achieved grand convergence. As noted, the country experienced the fastest decrease in child mortality in history.[47] Rwanda was considered a lost cause 25 years ago, with its broken economy and health system. The country was one of the poorest in the world, with a great burden of uncontrolled infectious diseases like tuberculosis, HIV/AIDS, and water-borne diseases. By 2014, premature mortality rates had dropped precipitously, and life expectancy had doubled.[48]

Another example is malaria bed nets, the focus of Chapter 8. In Tanzania, implementation scientists became involved with a local malaria bed net adoption program. By systematically accounting for factors that might influence the use of bed nets, they predicted that families were more concerned about the nuisance of being bitten by mosquitoes than they were of malaria.[49] While the governments' and donors' aims were to reduce malaria, they designed their campaign materials around promising families a peaceful night's sleep free from mosquito bites. They also demonstrated how the colour of the net affects its efficacy because nets lose effectiveness when frequently washed.[50] While whiter nets are cheaper (and therefore are the most commonly used colour), that choice can ultimately undercut the program's impact. Through implementation science, they leapfrogged over deep systemic and logistical challenges to get bed nets into the homes of millions of the most vulnerable across the region. Malaria is a leading cause of death in Africa. Fortunately, malaria control interventions, such as the use of insecticide-treated mosquito nets (ITNs, i.e., Malaria bed nets), have been shown to reduce the disease's burden significantly.[51,52] Sleeping under ITNs most nights, according to United Nations International Children's Emergency Fund,[53] is one of the most effective ways to prevent malaria morbidity and mortality. The use of malaria bed nets has reduced the number of children who die from malaria by 20%.[54] The Roll Back Malaria Program was launched in 1988, and many countries have made efforts since then to increase the coverage of this proven malaria control intervention.

Since 2000, external organization funding for malaria control in Africa has increased dramatically, reaching more than USD 1.47 billion in 2009.[55] As a result, across Africa, national coverage of the use of ITNs has increased drastically. Since 2000, over 1 billion ITNs have been distributed in Africa, and annual distribution is increasing.[53] Over 253 million ITNs were distributed to malaria-endemic countries in 2019.[53]

A study conducted by Eisele et al.[56] estimated that 831,100 deaths were prevented across 43 African countries by scaling up ITNs from 2001 to 2010. According to the study, Nigeria's ITN coverage increased from 0% to 45% between 2001 and 2010, preventing approximately 165,700 child malaria deaths.[56] Furthermore, a 10% increase in mosquito net ownership in Tanzania resulted in a 5.2% decrease in all-age malaria deaths.[57] Thus, increasing bed net ownership coverage will reduce malaria mortality. Based on UNICEF's report, most sub-Saharan African countries have made significant progress in household ownership of ITNs in recent years, with an average coverage of 69%. However, ownership of ITNs varies by country; for example, household ownership of ITNs is approximately 31% in Angola compared with 97% in Guinea-Bissau.[53]

We also see the importance of scaling up the COVID-19 vaccine. In Africa, by the beginning of 2022, less than 10% of the population had been fully vaccinated, marking the lowest rate globally. In comparison, by that time, half the world was fully vaccinated – countries like Canada and the United States had 77% and 63%, respectively, of their population fully vaccinated.[58] Limited funds and commodities, logistics, and travel costs have impacted the vaccine adoption process in the African region.[59] Storage requirements and regulatory hurdles for vaccines – lack of storage facilities, electricity, temperature regulation, and cold chain equipment – hampered the ability to store the vaccines safely, resulting in their expiration before use.[60]

Incorporating implementation science and scaling up evidence based on COVID-19 interventions in Africa can be highly effective in controlling the disease. Implementation science can help develop strategies to increase the acceptability, feasibility, adherence, and adoption of COVID-19 measures (physical distancing, use of masks) and the uptake of COVID-19 vaccines. Implementation research can be essential in assisting policymakers and public health departments in effectively designing and implementing pandemic response policies in their respective countries.[61]

Better training and software for data would help.[62] To increase vaccine adoption, demand for vaccines must rise, and supply needs to improve, but misinformation prevents people from taking the vaccine, resulting in low uptake. For example, like many African countries, Ghana was besieged by misinformation. At the start of 2022, Ghana had 7% of its population fully vaccinated. Ghana's Misinformation and Rumour Management Taskforce tried to combat this by working nationally and regionally to address false claims.[60]

Scaling Up Health Innovation Capacity in Africa and the Innovation Index

In 2020, the WHO developed a strategy to support the development and scale-up of innovative health solutions to improve health outcomes in Africa.[63] The Africa regional committee has reviewed and adopted this strategy to scale up health innovations in the African region.[63] The WHO Innovation Challenge, launched in October 2018, discovered about 2400 innovative solutions from 77 countries; 44 of these countries were in Africa.[64] This proved the continent's potential for developing innovations to address Africa's health challenges. Although international organizations are the primary investors for innovations in Africa, many African governments have made efforts to increase local and regional funding for scientific innovations. In 2015, the Developing Excellence in Leadership, Training and Science initiative was launched by the Wellcome Trust in partnership with the UK Department for International Development (DFID) and the Bill and Melinda Gates Foundation. The initiative aims to produce researchers who have the capacity to lead locally and conduct high-quality research to improve health and development, policy, and practice in Africa.[65] Also, the African Network for Drugs and Diagnostics Innovation focuses on coordinating existing research and development in Africa to address public health needs.[66]

According to the Global Innovation Index 2019, which examines global innovation growth and trends, high-income countries spend much more on research and development than LMICs.[67] In 2017, money spent on research and development was highest in North America (USD 1576 spent per person) and lowest in sub-Saharan Africa (USD 14.48 spent per person).[47] Sub-Saharan Africa ranks last in terms of innovation when compared with America, Europe, East Asia, and South and West Asia. According to Global Innovation Index 2021 reports for 132 countries worldwide, no African country made it to the top 50, and only four African countries – Mauritius, South Africa, Kenya, and Tanzania – made it to the top 100. Mauritius was ranked 51st, South Africa ranked 65th, Kenya ranked 85th, and the United Republic of Tanzania ranked 90th, while the top 10 countries are from Europe (Switzerland, the United Kingdom, and Sweden) and North America (the United States).[68]

Even though Africa accounts for 25% of the global disease burden, research and development pipelines to address diseases disproportionately affecting populations in Africa are insufficient. While Africa has 15% of the world's population, most of the countries in the continent spend less than 1% of their gross domestic product (GDP) on research and development.[69] The investment that does exist is primarily driven by the government, with a sizeable portion coming from international sources. The private sector's investment is limited primarily because of challenges with unstable political environments and corruption. For health innovation to thrive, collaborative and innovative financing mechanisms are required to support research and development in Africa.

African health innovators face numerous challenges in bringing their innovations to scale. According to a World Bank study,[69] African countries invest far less in innovation (approximately 0.01% per capita) than more advanced countries. For instance, in 2018, research and development expenditure (% of GDP) in the United Kingdom and the United States was 1.70% and 2.83%, respectively,[69] while for South Africa, the most innovative country in Africa, it was 0.75%. In 2019, Canada spent USD 36.6 billion on research and development, the United States spent USD 656.0 billion, and South Africa spent USD 2.44 billion.[69]

Aside from the lack of investment, the report revealed that most African countries also lack, to varying degrees, strong institutions, skilled human capital, appropriate infrastructure, technology, creative outputs, and market and business sophistication, all of which facilitate the scaling of innovations. The need is urgent to make funding and financing mechanisms available to African innovators, including access to capital.[70] Currently, programs like the African Network for Drugs and Diagnostics Innovation; the Alliance for Accelerating Excellence in Africa, developed by the African Academy of Sciences (AAS); and the New Partnership for Africa's Development (NEPAD) are African-led programs to support pan-African collaboration around scientific research and development.[37]

Additionally, African innovators experience difficulty with easily attaining a patent. The inability to patent an innovation can restrict

African innovators from transitioning their creation into a tangible business.[71] Factors stopping African innovators from attaining a patent include high legal costs, slow processing times, complex bureaucratic processes, and conflicting legislations between nations.[71] Teaching African innovators about the world of patents and organizations such as the World Intellectual Property Organization might be a move in the right direction.

NEPAD focuses on integrating existing technologies, fostering research and breakthrough discoveries, training and developing a science culture, and providing science and technology foresight through governance, regulation, and ethics.[72] In May 2020, the AAS announced its second Grand Challenges Africa Transition to Scale call. The call aims to support bold scientific innovations with the potential to provide long-term solutions to complex health and development challenges confronting African countries.

Implementation Science Training Capacity in Africa

The WHO has long been a leader in promoting health policy and systems research, including implementation research, with notable initiatives, including the 2011 report *Implementation Research for the Control of Infectious Diseases of Poverty*[73] and the 2012 publication of its first health policy and systems research strategy.[74] Furthermore, the WHO created *Implementation Research in Health: A Practical Guide* with the goal of increasing implementation science research capacity, particularly in LMICs.[75] The guide provides an introduction to basic implementation research concepts and language, briefly outlines what that entails, and describes the many exciting opportunities that it presents. The WHO support for implementation research continues with the publication of this guide.[75]

Implementation research requires multidisciplinary teams to use specialized skills to clarify the implementation context, engage key partners, design theory- and partner-informed interventions, and conduct rigorous theory-based evaluations in real-world settings. As a result, establishing Implementation science research capacity requires training to obtain these unique skills. Such training is primarily available in Europe and North America, although growing efforts are expanding in LMICs, especially in Africa.[76] Most training programs in North America and Europe are out of reach for most trainees from resource-poor countries because of the high costs. Although implementation science training programs are expanding in Africa, opportunities remain limited, and costs associated with international or regional travel can be prohibitive for many trainees. While online options exist, many still emphasize didactic content over personalized mentorship, although newer models are increasingly incorporating mentorship to support the successful initiation and completion of implementation science projects. Addressing Africa's health challenges may necessitate a significant investment in implementation science research to bridge the gap between evidence and practice.

Implementation science research is required to scale up evidence-based interventions for sickle cell disease management in Africa to reduce the pain, morbidity, and premature death it causes.[77] Most individuals with sickle cell disease are born in Africa, with up to 3% of births in the African continent being affected by the disease.[78,79] Sickle cell disease is rare in Europe and North America. Despite the evidence-based healthcare interventions that have been effective in reducing morbidity and mortality, approximately 50% to 90% of children with sickle cell disease born in Africa die before the age of 10.[79,80] Africa lacks a multifaceted implementation strategy that explores the uptake and long-term sustainability of evidence-based interventions for sickle cell disease[77] and would require robust training programs to build capacity in the implementation of sickle cell disease management.

Several universities promote implementation science in Africa; some of these universities teach implementation science and offer scholarships for implementation science programs. The implementation science program at Stellenbosch University in South Africa is available full-time for a minimum of one year and part-time for a minimum of two years. As part of the Kenya AIDS Vaccine Initiative-Institute of Clinical Research mandate to build capacity, a doctor of philosophy (PhD) degree in implementation science is offered at the University of Nairobi. In 2021, the University of the Witwatersrand in South Africa invited qualified candidates to apply for a full-time funded master's degree program in implementation science. The Special Programme for Research and Training in Tropical Diseases[81] advances effective and innovative global health research and is co-sponsored by UNICEF, United Nations Development Programme, the World Bank, and the WHO. The scheme's goal is to increase graduate training capacity in implementation research and the number of researchers in LMICs. The University of Nairobi has also developed a training program to build local capacity for implementation science with support from the Medical Education Partnership Initiative of the Vanderbilt Institute for Global Health.[76] The curriculum content includes core theory, methods, and experiences in implementation science. The program employs a team mentoring and supervision approach, with fellows matched with mentors from the University of Nairobi and partnering institutions, including the University of Washington in Seattle and the University of Maryland.[76]

Several research centres and institutes promote implementation science in Africa; for example, the Implementation Research Division of the Aurum Institute conducts health research and scientific evaluations for HIV and tuberculosis prevention, care, and treatment. This institute employs a wide range of disciplines, including epidemiology, biostatistics, health policy, health economics, management sciences, sociology, psychology, and others, to identify, develop, and assess the impact of innovative HIV and tuberculosis service delivery strategies.[82] It also concentrates on hospitals, communities, correctional facilities, and mines. It conducts scientific research on issues relating to implementing policies, programs, or practices that contribute to national, regional, and global strategies and goals. By incorporating research methodology into program implementation, the institute uses implementation research to improve the quality, efficiency, and effectiveness of service delivery strategies.[82]

In addition, the Center for Translation and Implementation Research (CTAIR) in Nigeria, operating under the College of Medicine at the University of Nigeria, provides external funding to university faculty for translation and implementation research. CTAIR focuses on advancing research, skill training, and community training to promote public health in Africa through implementation science.[83] The Nigerian Implementation Science Alliance emerged in 2015[84] with the aim of advancing healthcare through implementation science and research. It actively identifies and disseminates implementation research to partners across Nigeria, collaborating with over 50 organizations and four multi-centre research teams.[85]

The Africa Academy for Public Health (AAPH) is dedicated to innovative scientific research, training, and capacity building for healthcare managers and providers.[86] The institute offers short courses in implementation science and health economic evaluation, with an emphasis on HIV prevention and treatment.[86] The course aims to teach students how to describe and critically discuss major concepts and evaluate academic studies in implementation science and health economics and use key mathematical estimators and approaches commonly used in implementation science and health economics.[86] Through the Africa Research Implementation Science and Education network, the next generation of leaders in public health implementation science and health system research in Africa are trained. The network also provides training opportunities to advance mastery of both new knowledge (implementation of health system interventions, health service quality, health systems financing, human resources for health) and methods (implementation science, program and impact evaluations, biostatistics and epidemiology, and health economics).[86] Furthermore, through rigorous coursework, participatory seminars, case studies, intensive mentorship, and training in translational research, trainees have the opportunity to interact extensively with faculty, fellow trainees, and other professional mentors.[86]

The Africa Early Childhood Network (AfECN) strengthens research network capacity by mentoring research teams to deepen early childhood development research programs that are related to policy and practices in various regions of Africa.[87] It also advances policy and program research by documenting best practices and improving communication among scholars and between scholars and the government, society, and non-governmental organizations (NGOs). Recognizing the insufficiency of relevant empirical evidence required to guide program design and implementation, AfECN works to support African scholars working at the intersection of research, practice, and policy to advance early childhood development in the region. AfECN also facilitates a regional research network that brings together well-known global early childhood development scholars from both within and outside the region to improve knowledge generation, management, and dissemination.[87]

The Global Research on Implementation and Translation Science (GRIT) consortium was established in 2018.[88] With projects spanning eight countries – Ghana, Guatemala, India, Kenya, Vietnam, Malawi, Nepal, and Rwanda – GRIT is dedicated to strengthening research and training infrastructure in dissemination and implementation for improved hypertension care. All eight GRIT members have capacity building activities in the following areas: (1) tools, (2) skills, (3) staff and infrastructure, and (4) structure, systems, and roles, based on the Potter and Brough capacity pyramid.[89] The greatest number of activities are in the skills and tools section, which are more technical (versus sociocultural) and easier to implement.[90] In 2019, the Central and West Africa Implementation Science Alliance (CAWISA) was established to target Nigeria, Cameroon, the Democratic Republic of the Congo, and Ghana. CAWISA's five-point plan prioritizes leadership and vision, research productivity and impact, scholars and mentors, strategic partnerships, and sustained funding.[91]

This book discusses 10 evidence-based innovations. Chapter 2 focuses on ORS, which cost very little and can reduce deaths from childhood diarrhea by over 90%, but are accessible to only 4 out of 10 children who need them, and what can be done to improve these numbers in Africa. Chapter 3 explores seven significant factors in enhancing handwashing in Africa, drawing from several innovative water, sanitation, and hygiene programs and other sanitation programs in the region. Chapter 4 centres on the drug praziquantel, used in preventative chemotherapy, for schistosomiasis, a neglected tropical disease, and the challenges to implementation with a focus on its administration in Nigeria. Drawing from several case studies, Chapter 5 discusses the application of biotech in agriculture and how trust plays an essential and multifaceted role in scaling it up. Chapter 6 provides strategies for improving vitamin A supplementation in Africa, particularly in light of the rapid decline in the COVID-19 pandemic. With the ubiquity of mobile phones in Africa, mobile health (mHealth) has become a more effective means of developing services, which is the topic covered in Chapter 7, using MomConnect as the innovation of focus. Chapter 8 deals with malaria bed nets and implementation science's role in leapfrogging over profound systemic and logistical challenges and navigating cultural complexities. Chapter 9 draws attention to polio eradication and what might be needed to reach the finish line. The Meningitis Vaccine Project (MVP), a very successful vaccination program in Burkina Faso and along the Meningitis Belt, is the focus of Chapter 10. Chapter 11 explores the human papillomavirus (HPV) vaccination campaign, a success story in Rwanda with exceptional results. Finally, in Chapter 12, drawing from these innovations, I summarize key considerations for policymakers and interested parties within the field of implementation science.

Health innovations can improve many individuals' lives in Africa, from disease prevention to healthier lifestyles. Although implementation science plays a crucial role in scaling up these innovations, the many barriers it faces in supporting the impact these innovations can have on health must be recognized and addressed. Technological advances and promotion of implementation science training in Africa have assisted this process. However, government health ministries and global health funders need to prioritize implementation science research to maximize the scale and reach of health innovations in the region to save and improve more lives.

2
The ORS Paradox: Why the Gap and What to Do about It

The discovery that sodium transport and glucose transport are coupled in the small intestine so that glucose accelerates absorption of solute and water was potentially the most important medical advance [of the twentieth] century.

– *The Lancet*, 5 August 1978

Diarrhea is a leading killer of children, with hundreds of thousands of children dying every year. These deaths are nearly entirely preventable if sick children receive proper diarrheal treatment. The treatment is based on a discovery more than 50 years old – ORS. According to *The Lancet*,[92] the profound implications of understanding the coupling of sodium and glucose transport in the small intestine was a pivotal medical discovery in the last century and paved the way for the development of ORS, helping save countless lives by treating dehydration, particularly for diarrhea-related cases. However, ORS, which costs just pennies and can avert most of these deaths, reaches only 4 out of 10 children who need them.

This chapter focuses on the history, development, challenges, and implementation and scaling strategies of ORS treatments in Africa from 1981 to 2020. It analyzes critical barriers to the adoption of ORS in the region and facilitators and potential solutions to ensure wider reach and effectiveness.

What exactly is ORS? It is a solution that helps treat dehydration from diarrhea and replenish the body with lost fluids and electrolytes. It contains three main ingredients: clean water, electrolytes/salts, and carbohydrates (usually sugar). In 1969, a balanced glucose-electrolyte mixture was created and used by the WHO and UNICEF.[93] In 1984, a standard ORS version was created with trisodium citrate instead of sodium bicarbonate to improve ORS stability in hot climates, which contained 90 mEq/L of sodium with a total osmolarity of 311 mOsm/L. Then in 2001, a reduced osmolarity version of ORS, also known as new ORS, was created to increase safety and efficacy in children, with a reduction in its sodium concentration to 75 mEq/L, glucose concentration to 75 mmol/L, and total osmolarity to 245 mOsm/L.[93]

History of ORS

The standard ORS was initially discovered in the 1970s by Dilip Mahalanabis, when the need for a solution to life-threatening diarrhea was high, and rehydration through intravenous (IV) solutions could not meet the demands of the thousands of individuals in developing nations.[94] The lack of sterile solutions in countries with few medical resources or sanitary conditions made IV rehydration solutions less feasible, and thus a need for a more practical solution that considered the social environment became important.[94]

The introduction of the standard ORS by Mahalanabis built on decades of iterative discoveries. For example, in 1949, Dr. Daniel Darrow first advocated for the earliest types of ORS, before the standard ORS, which contained potassium, sodium chloride, and glucose, based on observations of which electrolytes the body lost during diarrhea.[95] Dr. Darrow was a research physician at Yale University and served as the resident of the American Pediatrics Association in 1959.[96] These earliest types of ORS reduced case fatality rates of babies from dehydration to less than 5%; however, he could not ascertain the right concentrations for each electrolyte. Using what was known from Dr. Darrow's discovery, the next major observation that led to the development of ORS was in 1953, when sugar physiologists R. B. Fisher and D. S. Parsons discovered part of the glucose transport mechanism in the small intestine, which has sites for specific receptors associated with it.[95] This discovery showed the mechanism by which glucose was absorbed, which helped to better explain rehydration therapy.[95] In 1958, this work was expanded on by physiologists Emanuel Rikilis and Juda Hirsch Quastel, who studied in Imperial College and worked at McGill University.[97] These researchers showed that active absorption of glucose in a Guinea pig's intestines depended on sodium (Na) ions and worked on determining optimal concentrations for water, sodium, and glucose absorption.[95] Another sugar physiologist, Robert Crane, then defined the mechanism for active transport of glucose when Na was present.[95]

Combined, these studies helped develop the appropriate concentrations of each substance for future ORS.[95] In the late 1950s, Drs. Curran, Schultz, and Zalusky found that glucose absorption in the small intestine required luminal Na and that Na absorption was enhanced with luminal glucose in rabbits.[94] This was important because sodium and sugar were absorbed together by a particular protein; thus, creating a solution that contained sodium, like ORS, would facilitate glucose absorption.[94] Wright and colleagues later identified the intestinal glucose-Na transporter as SGLT1.[94] Another major observation was that cholera (a disease that induces severe diarrhea) enterotoxin (cyclic AMP) did not inhibit Na that was stimulated by glucose; therefore, fluid absorption still occurred.[94] This discovery showed that cholera-toxin-mediated cyclic AMP secretion did not affect glucose-induced Na absorption because glucose did not require cyclic AMP to stimulate Na absorption. This was important because it demonstrated that ORS works well because of independent absorptive and secretory processes.[94]

In 1961, when the cholera pandemic started in the Philippines, Dr. Robert A. Phillips found that adding glucose to electrolyte solutions increased sodium absorption, as rehydrating with just water was not enough to replenish the lost water and salt from diarrhea.[95] This led to the development of a clinical trial that Phillips and Lieutenant Commander Craig Wallace conducted for patients with diarrhea. Of 30 patients, 5 died after receiving ORS because of the improper concentrations of electrolytes. This encouraged other researchers to continue to assess the correct concentrations to allow optimal absorption of Na.[95] The last important event was the use of ORS by Dilip Mahalanabis in the Bangladeshi War of Independence in the early 1970s.[94] It was administered to people with cholera in refugee camps in Bengal, where they were provided with bags of salt and sugar in water, based on the pre-standard version of ORS.[98] Case fatality ratios from cholera and other diarrheal disease dropped below 4%, compared with the original 30%.[98]

Finally in 1978, the WHO created the diarrheal disease control program that popularized standard ORS (created in 1984 with trisodium citrate) for worldwide use.[98]

Refining ORS

Since ORS is a low-cost health technology, as presented by the UNICEF Child Survival Revolution, it led to a collaboration between the WHO and UNICEF, along with the Control for Diarrheal Diseases (CDD) program, to combine financial assets, produce ORS, and support various countries. Other bilateral agencies, such as the US Agency for International Development (USAID), also prioritized CDD and provided much support to countries' programs.[99] Between 1980 and 1995, the CDD conducted research to assess the aetiology and epidemiology of childhood diarrhea. This research also included a re-evaluation of the standard ORS formulation from the 1970s, which used 111 mmol/L glucose, 90 mmol/L sodium, 30 mmol/L bicarbonate, 20 mmol/L potassium, and 80 mmol/L chloride.[99] In the 1980s, 30 mmol/L sodium bicarbonate was replaced by 10 mmol/L tri-sodium citrate, which created more stable, cheaper, and simply packaged ORS contents.[100,101] Then in the 1990s, over 50 studies evaluated differences between the standard citrate ORS and experimental formulations based on glycine, L-alanine, L-glutamine, maltodextrin, and rice to enhance absorption; however, none were found to be more effective than standard citrate ORS.[102] As more studies were conducted, it was found that reducing the osmolarity of ORS, and thereby lowering the glucose and sodium concentrations, would reduce stool output, vomiting, and IV therapy.[103] This lower osmolarity ORS was then recommended by the WHO in 2002.[103]

ORS has been promoted as an essential medicine to treat diarrhea by the WHO and UNICEF. The WHO began a global initiative to increase ORS usage in 1978. The campaign's activities included an educational program, public awareness, and health worker training. In July 2019, the WHO added co-packaged ORS and zinc to its list of essential medications for children, aligning with best practices for diarrhea treatment.[104] The WHO recommends oral zinc (tablets or syrups) as adjunct therapy with ORS for acute childhood diarrhea. Zinc supplements help to restore levels of the micronutrient, and mixing zinc with ORS can be an attractive approach for simultaneous provision of these two effective interventions. In contrast to ORS, there are variations of homemade rehydration solutions, alternatively known as recommended home fluids. These are essentially non-packaged home fluids such as cereal-salt, rice-water or sugar-salt solutions,[105] as well as other common home fluids such as juice or tea.[106]

The ORS Delivery Gap

Death resulting from diarrhea is caused by the rapid loss of bodily fluids, which leads to dehydration and malnutrition. However, the intestinal absorption of glucose and sodium can continue during a diarrhea episode, which offers an avenue for rehydration to match this sudden loss of fluids and recovery. Focusing on this mechanism, ORS has become the standard treatment for diarrhea in children.

Why is ORS, which costs just pennies and reduces deaths from childhood diarrhea by over 90%,[14] reaching only an average of 4 in 10 affected children? We know that ORS interventions work, but despite the simplicity of this intervention, less than half of the children who need it receive the treatment. Even in countries with sound diarrhea treatment policies, there have been gaps between policy and implementation. The varied and low uptake of ORS intervention programming underscores the importance of understanding what factors influence the accessibility and scaling of treatment.

Guidelines for ORS were established in 1980, and the CDD helped develop pharmaceutical facilities for LMICs to create ORS packages.[99] The CDD was created by the WHO in 1978 to reduce diarrhea-related mortality among infants and children in developing nations.[107] The program focused on reducing mortality through case management with specific clinical management guidelines, including prevention or treatment of dehydration with ORS, feeding and breastfeeding during a diarrhea episode, and using antibiotics only in bloody diarrhea cases.[108] CDD managers training courses were held in 1983 and were attended by 170 individuals from 49 countries.[109] Promotional and educational materials were distributed to 43 countries to encourage ORS uptake and demonstrate its importance.[109] UNICEF and the WHO helped manufacture ORS.[109]

Guidelines for production were monitored and revised in 1985 and 2005 to ensure optimal quality and reflect changes in ORS concentration values.[99] In 1993, 60 developing countries were creating satisfactory ORS packets. In 1995, about 80% of diarrhea cases had access to ORS and 34% were using ORT.[99] By the end of 1995, over 7300 courses had been held and over 570,000 health workers had been trained.[99] This meant approximately 38% of health workers were trained to treat children with diarrhea.[99]

The big question remains: how do we reach the other 6 out of 10 children who need ORS, especially the significant proportion who reside in Africa?

As of 2019, high-income countries have decreased diarrheal disease–related mortality rates (0.73% of total prevalent cases), compared with LMICs (2.02% of total prevalent cases).[110] Currently, ORS has a global coverage of only 43%; therefore, more than half of the individuals who need it are not receiving it.[111] Global ORS implementation has plateaued over the past few decades because of poor political commitment, low resources, and lack of community understanding and awareness.[112] Challenges to implementation also include ORS supply, cost, taste, and clean water accessibility.[113] Though inequality in ORS coverage decreased from 2000 to 2017 between countries, including Central African Republic, Mongolia, Myanmar, and Sierra Leone, within countries, geographical inequalities still prevent certain areas from receiving ORS treatment.[106] In 2017, about 6,519,000 children with diarrhea were not treated with ORS.[106]

Scaling Up of ORS in Africa

Diarrhea disease is a significant public health concern; the WHO reports that the disease is the second-leading cause of death in children under five.[114] Despite the inclusion of ORS in the WHO Essential Medicines List and Global Action Plan for the prevention and control of pneumonia and diarrhea, the coverage of ORS remains low, especially in African countries like Mali, Togo, and Senegal.[115] A study on the progress of ORS coverage highlights major reasons why the scale-up of ORS coverage has stagnated.[116] These reasons include a lack of political commitment, insufficient ORS supplies, poor ORS distribution, a lack of awareness of ORS use, and inadequate health worker training.[116] Also, a systematic review of studies on the implementation of ORS identified factors that promote ORS coverage.[117] These factors include the availability and accessibility of ORS, as well as community members' awareness and education about ORS and the free distribution of ORS in communities.

ORS coverage is highest in southern sub-Saharan Africa and lowest in central, western, and eastern sub-Saharan Africa.[106] In Africa, various methods have been used to scale up ORS implementation. In Senegal, USAID's "technical assistance" programs were executed in the country to introduce ORS through "health huts" and community care management.[118] Some barriers to ORS implementation in Senegal included weak distribution systems; low knowledge of ORS; cost and reliance on external funders; private pharmacies, which may under-prescribe ORS; and substitution with homemade solutions.[113,119] In contrast, Sierra Leone is highly successful in its ORS implementation because of strong community-based support for ORS treatment, and volunteers are trained to promote hygiene practice and treat diarrhea with ORT.[113] Other areas, such as Mali, promote ORS through radio, television, and child survival interventions; however, it is mostly considered along with other therapies because of time and monetary restraints and the knowledge that ORS cannot prevent diarrhea reoccurrence.[120,121] Therefore, improving future interventions informed by these barriers and facilitators may improve ORS implementation in Africa.

Several international organizations, NGOs, and the governments of many African countries have made efforts to scale up the use of ORS in African countries since its recommendation by the WHO for the treatment of diarrhea. The Blue Flag volunteers in Sierra Leone were trained to treat diarrhea with ORT even before the civil war. After the civil war, the primary healthcare system of the country was reinvented, and repeated diarrhea outbreaks were treated with ORS, as recommended by the government.[106] The Sierra Leone government ensured that the supply chain for ORS was maintained at all levels, as accessibility to ORS is a critical facilitator for its use.[117] To ensure that ORS was available, the Ministry of Health intensified its tracking efforts. Blue Flag volunteers and community-based distributors publicized ORS in various districts and communities throughout Sierra Leone, ensuring that people were aware of the intervention. In 2010, the government of Sierra Leone launched the Free Health Care Initiative. This initiative eliminated healthcare user fees for pregnant women, nursing mothers, and children under the age of five.[122] According to Wiens et al.,[106] while Sierra Leone had increased ORS coverage in 2000, the pace was gradual until 2010, when health costs for children and pregnant and lactating women were abolished. The Free Health Care Initiative increased healthcare use, which resulted in the scale-up of ORS in the country.[123]

Several programs and initiatives have been developed by the USAID in Senegal since 1985; these initiatives include PRITECH, BASICS, and the Child Survival Program.[118] UNICEF was the sole provider of ORS in Senegal until 2000. USAID and UNICEF supplied ORS to the country's Ministry of Health, and the drug was given free.[118]

The government of Malawi implemented the CDD initiative in I985. UNICEF supplied large quantities of ORS packets, which were distributed to all health facilities in the country.[124] The government ensured that ORS packets were widely available in healthcare organizations. ORS was the standard treatment for diarrhea in nearly all health services, including hospitals, across the nation. The Malawi Ministry of Health Education Service was incorporated into the CDD program to ensure the general public was well versed in ORS intervention. Most healthcare facilities in Malawi had areas for ORT administration and education.[124] Furthermore, USAID supported Population Services International (PSI) in socially marketing branded ORS in Malawi; as a result of this initiative, ORS is widely used and recognized in Malawi.[106] The Malawian government also ensured that ORS was accessible to everybody by making it free in the public sector and subsidized in the private sector.[125]

In 2012, the Federal Ministry of Health of Nigeria and the National Primary Health Care Development Agency launched the Essential Childhood Medicines Scale-Up Plan: 2012–2015. This was the first national initiative for reducing child mortality by promoting access to life-saving treatments like ORS.[126] With funding from the Norwegian Agency for Development Cooperation and Global Affairs Canada, the Clinton Health Access Initiative (CHAI) supported the Nigerian government in implementing a program that aligned with the Essential Childhood Medicines Scale-Up Plan's strategies and activities between 2013 and 2017. This initiative included strategies to promote universal availability and affordability of ORS in eight states (Bauchi, Cross River, Lagos, Kaduna, Kano, Katsina, Niger, and Rivers) in the country.[127]

ORS Implementation Lessons in Africa

In a systematic review, key barriers and facilitators to ORS were uncovered from 55 articles published between 1981 and 2020.[117] Twenty-two of these studies were focused on Africa, and the key factors to scaling ORS revolved around four broad vital areas: (1) availability and accessibility, (2) knowledge, (3) partnership engagement, and (4) design and acceptability.

Availability and Accessibility

Availability and accessibility can be understood both as barriers and as facilitators depending on the equitable distribution and reliability of supplies. If a program is going to offer ORS, it needs to get to the people that need it most, on time, and consistently. Costs can also prohibit uptake. If you want to save lives, make it affordable. It doesn't matter how great it is, if people can't pay for it, they won't use it.

Egypt was one of the first countries to administer ORS at the national level, and its experience is a great public success story. The National Control of Diarrheal Disease Project (NCDDP) was founded in 1981 in conjunction with USAID. By 1984, the program was fully operating across the country.[128] The project aimed to lower diarrheal mortality in children under five by at least 25%. The principal strategy employed was uninterrupted supply and distribution of ORS.[128] Chemical Industries Development, a government-owned corporation, was primarily responsible for ORS production. The company sold ORS packets to NCDDP, which then distributed the ORS packets to the public and private sectors at a subsidized rate. Throughout the project, a comprehensive tracking system was created to aid in projecting demand and achieving the project's goal of continuous supply. By 1985, ORS production had almost doubled from 4.5 million litres in 1981 to 8.6 million litres.[128] The private and public sectors were actively engaged in the distribution of ORS in Egypt. During the program, it was observed that the distance between homes and health centres made it difficult for people in rural areas to obtain and use ORS. According to Wilson et al.,[113] distance, cost, and money required for transportation are significant barriers to the use of ORS in rural areas. Thus, keeping the cost of ORS low can make the product more accessible.[113] To address this issue and ensure that ORS is available and accessible in more remote rural areas in Egypt, NCDDP recruited about 3000 depot holders to store ORS packets in their houses and distribute them to villagers for a low price (roughly two cents) or for free.[129] The depot holders, who included community leaders, traditional birth attendants, and health workers, were trained to use ORS. During the project, private sector distribution posed a significant challenge because ORS had to compete with more profitable anti-diarrheal drugs. To address this issue, the NCDDP created financial incentives for pharmacies and chemist stores to promote ORS. Pharmacies were given free measuring cups, which they could sell along with ORS packets.[130]

The *British Medical Journal* termed the NCDDP "the world's most successful program. The number of diarrheal deaths in infants and children under the age of five had dropped by nearly two-thirds, while diarrheal deaths as a percentage of all deaths among children under the age of five had dropped from 45 percent to 28 percent" by the end of the program.[128(p.12)]

Even if ORS is known, the scaling up of ORS is impossible if the product is not available and accessible. Once universal familiarity with ORS is achieved, availability is essential. One of the strategies adopted by CHAI to scale up the use of ORS in eight states in Nigeria between 2012 and 2017 was "market shaping." CHAI aimed to make affordable, high-quality ORS and zinc more widely available in those states.[131] To promote ORS manufacturing in the country, CHAI worked with local manufacturers to encourage investments in the production, promotion, and sale of high-quality ORS products. Also, market intelligence on Nigeria's demand was provided to suppliers, as well as one-on-one technical advice on product registration, cost reduction, and marketing strategies.[127] Through this support, four new low-osmolarity ORS, and seven co-packaged ORS and zinc products were introduced into the Nigerian market.

In addition to providing support to manufacturers, CHAI collaborated with Nigeria's National Agency for Food and Drug Administration and Control (NAFDAC) to persuade suppliers to transition to a low-osmolarity ORS formulation. Before the program, the Nigerian market already had 21 ORS products.[127] However, there was only one low-osmolarity ORS registered in the nation; by the end of the program,

NAFDAC had registered 35 low-osmolarity ORS. In addition, CHAI worked with Nigeria's entire private-sector supply chain to expand the availability of ORS and zinc in rural areas. To achieve this, innovative private sector strategies and streamlined distribution models targeting wholesalers, sub-distributors, and retailers were adopted.[127] Stationed brand-agnostic marketers were placed at wholesale outlets to provide educational materials and persuade private retailers to sell ORS. The private sector's market-shaping efforts resulted in a significant increase in ORS and zinc sales in the country. Private suppliers' sales of ORS increased from 7.1 million units in 2014 to 27.1 million units in 2016.[131]

In Sierra Leone, ORS was widely accessible, thanks to the supply chain management in both the public and private sectors.[113] Similarly, the high availability of ORS in both sectors contributed to Malawi's successful implementation of ORS use.[113]

A well-organized group of community-based distributors can greatly extend the reach of the public health sector to achieve a market penetration scale. Support should be provided to the private sector to identify a clear path towards the creation of a sustainable market for ORS.

The government and partners must seek to reduce the cost of ORS in African countries, where it is still prohibitively expensive for the majority of people.[113] The government and its partners must ensure that ORS packets are available in rural areas at a reasonable cost. ORS packets should be distributed to various outlets in rural areas. The free distribution of ORS through primary care providers also facilitates its use in the community, particularly in rural areas. Wagner et al.[132] confirm that free and convenient distribution increased ORS coverage.

In April 2010, Sierra Leone's president launched the Free Health Care Initiative for pregnant women, nursing mothers, and children under five.[133] Earlier data from the Ministry of Sanitation and Health had revealed that financial costs were a major barrier to mothers and children seeking healthcare in Sierra Leone.[133] The use of ORS in the country has also increased as a result of this initiative, according to evidence.[113]

Knowledge

Low knowledge of ORS treatments and where and how to access those treatments was observed to be a barrier to overall ORS implementation. However, this barrier was remediated and became a facilitator to the implementation of ORS when information was readily shared between multiple interested parties and healthcare professionals, researchers, patients, and family members, and they all participated in the discussion.

Educating the public on the causes of childhood diarrhea and the significance of ORS is necessary for increasing its uptake. Furthermore, knowledge of ORS can be improved through social marketing and educational campaigns that inform the public about the product's availability and increase knowledge and confidence regarding proper product preparation and administration.[134]

As early as 1992, 90% of Malawian moms who had given birth in the previous five years were aware of ORS.[135] This was due to advertising at health facilities and information, education, and communication programs using newspapers, a Ministry of Health circular called *Moyo Magazine*, and radio jingles.[135] PSI, with USAID's support, began a global marketing campaign to promote its ORS brand Thanzi in 1999.[125] According to a 2004 evaluation of PSI's social marketing work, Thanzi was "advertised and promoted via branded and generic radio advertisements, posters, mobile video shows, and theater shows."[135(p.3),125] A survey conducted just two years after Thanzi's launch discovered that 79% of respondents had heard of the product, and 85% of the respondents correctly identified its function.[125] The majority of Malawi moms stated they learned about ORS from the Malawi Broadcasting Corporation and community health professionals.[136] From 2005 onward, PSI continued to market its Thanzi brand using mass media and interpersonal communications.[135] In 2005 and 2008, PSI conducted national tracking surveys to modify its strategy. By 2010, 96% of Malawian mothers were familiar with the Thanzi brand.[137] Therefore, using mass media will help to facilitate the determinants of ORS use. Kenya et al.[138] also confirm that a combination of a commercial approach and mass communication technique could increase knowledge of ORS.

ORT corners were implemented in health facilities in Bauchi and Sokoto states in Nigeria. The ORT Corners serve as treatment centres for sick children and provide caregivers with the knowledge and skills required to manage diarrhea episodes and prevent diarrhea.[139] Evidence shows that the ORT Corners implemented in these states played a significant role in diarrhea management. ORT Corner users had a better understanding of ORS than non-Corner users. They also demonstrated the ability to manage diarrhea at home, compared with ORT Corner non-users.[139]

In Burundi, diarrhea is the major cause of death among children under the age of five, accounting for 18% of all deaths.[140] From 2004, as part of a USAID-funded program to minimize childhood morbidity and mortality, PSI/Burundi has been supplying ORS through commercial shops in Burundi under the brand ORASEL (a low-osmolarity ORS product developed by FDC Limited and branded and distributed by

PSI).[141] Despite these efforts, a nationally representative baseline survey of female caregivers of children under the age of five, done in 2006, revealed that only 20% of carers had given their children ORASEL during the child's most recent diarrhea episode.[141] Based on these findings, PSI/Burundi implemented a variety of social marketing strategies to improve ORASEL use, including public demonstrations on how to prepare and use it, distribution of print and radio messages about ORASEL's benefits, and changing the taste from bitter to orange.[140] Two radio spots focused on the importance and use of ORS, while the other two focused on the causes and consequences of diarrhea, particularly the severity of diarrhea in children and how to prevent it.[134] These adverts were aired 4994 times on six radio stations. In addition, community outreach initiatives were held in schools and health centres to complement the radio program. The impact of the effort was determined by an evaluation survey conducted in 2007.[141] The use of ORASEL had increased to 30% among all caregivers; among those who had been highly exposed to the PSI campaign, 75% had treated their child with ORASEL during the child's most recent diarrhea episode. Furthermore, caregivers who were highly exposed to the campaign had significantly higher knowledge of using ORASEL (from 28% at baseline to 88% at follow-up). In another study, less than half of all caregivers could adequately prepare homemade ORS.[142] These findings overall show that ORS social marketing and skill-building interventions could help caregivers use ORS more effectively. Knowledge of ORS and use patterns are better in urban areas, as most people there are more educated than in rural areas, where the majority of those with no formal education dwell.[105]

Partnership and Engagement

Partnership engagement centred on buy-in and the trustworthiness of the ORS program, which ultimately needed to be there from day one to enable scaling and implementation. Social and mass media were observed to be a great tool for increasing awareness of program availability, which helped families learn what ORS treatment was and where this treatment was located. The role of local governments cannot be understated as a critical partner in the promotion and support of ORS programs, as without this relationship, ORS programs' sustainability was severely limited.

Local communities and key participants should initiate partnerships, have a better understanding of nuanced challenges and cultural barriers within local geographies, and be equipped to provide advice and support change. A combination of expanding manufacturing and distribution of ORS and the training of healthcare professionals is beneficial for increasing ORS uptake.[117]

The USAID's mission in Ghana invited Strengthening Health Outcomes through the Private Sector (SHOPS) to execute a comprehensive program in Ghana to increase the availability and usage of ORS.[143] The program's initial design of robust public partnerships contributed to its success. First, SHOPS partnered with local pharmaceutical companies (such as M&G Pharmaceuticals, LaGray Chemicals, and Phyto-Riker) to manufacture and market ORS and zinc products in the country. This partnership led to the production of Zintab (zinc tablets) and Hydralate (an ORS) in Ghana.[143]

Also, as frontline providers in the community, drug retailers and over-the-counter-medical sellers (OTCMS) were engaged in the program implementation. Despite their vital role in rural areas, SHOPS observed that shop assistants and OTCMS do not have formal drug-dispensing training. Recognizing this, SHOPS proposed a partnership with the Ghana Pharmacy Council, which conducts the annual training required for OTCMS re-accreditation. The Pharmacy Council trained about 8000 OTCMS and 1500 pharmacists in Ghana, thanks to SHOPS' support. Recognizing the strength of Ghana's private provider network, SHOPS expanded the diarrhea management training to include midwives and other technicians, in addition to drug store owners and assistants. SHOPS partnered with the Association of Community Pharmacists, Ghana Registered Midwives Association, and Ghana Physician Assistants Association to train 1159 extra private sector providers, including pharmacy technicians, dispensing technicians, and physician assistants. SHOPS also collaborated with two NGOs (Health Keepers and Precision Development Xperts) to design a diarrhea management training module for community distribution agents. According to a 2012 randomized controlled study, 66% of trained OTCMS sold ORS and zinc to secret shoppers.[143]

SHOPS also partnered with the Ghana Behavior Change Support (BCS) project to raise awareness of ORS. The objectives were to incorporate messages about ORS into the BCS Good Life umbrella campaign, which created and broadcasted media messages on a variety of health topics, and to develop a targeted national mass media campaign to introduce ORS and promote its use in the treatment of pediatric diarrhea.[143]

SHOPS' robust partnership strategy was the main determinant in successfully increasing the availability and use of ORS in Ghana. SHOPS' strategic alliances with local manufacturers maintained a steady supply of high-quality diarrhea treatment items for both the public and private sectors. Close engagement with Ghana's Ministry of Health and other regulatory bodies (Pharmacy Council, Food and Drug Authority) facilitated product provider training and the quick registration of new products. Recognition and engagement with OTCMS as community front-line providers was a fantastic initiative that was critical to increasing ORS use in Ghana because OTCMS are frequently the first point of contact for caregivers looking for critical medications, particularly in remote locations. However, despite their significance, OTCMS are frequently disregarded. SHOPS' recognition of and engagement with OTCMS was a brilliant strategy.

A similar package of interventions with robust partnerships can be applied in other African regions to scale up the use of ORS.

CHAI partnered with the Nigerian government to implement a program in eight states to expand the use of ORS and zinc in diarrhea treatment.[131] Healthcare providers in both the public and private sectors were engaged in the program. To involve the healthcare community, multiple channels and platforms were used, including state-level training, supportive supervision, CME sessions, and professional associations. A similar multichannel approach was used to involve community members in the eight states. Local manufacturers of ORS were also engaged in the program to encourage investments in the production, promotion, and sales of ORS.[131] Informal providers, such as chemists, were educated on the role of ORS, and they were encouraged to prescribe ORS to patients suffering from diarrhea.

Engagement of commercial providers and participation of non-government organizations and the private and public sector are instrumental in improving ORS uptake.

Design and Acceptability

Finally, the design and acceptability of ORS highlighted that local community-driven initiatives are more effective. Locals will help design a program that works best for them. It is important to listen and include them at all levels of program design, implementation, and scaling. These local participants have a deeper grasp of the various subtle difficulties and cultural barriers that exist within local geographies. They may also offer advice and assistance for implementing designs to overcome these obstacles.

The packaging of a product is equally crucial to its implementation. When ORS is packaged separately or in pouches with zinc, all with instructional messaging for the intended user, it increases the use of ORS. In Ethiopia, to increase the use and implementation of ORS, zinc was co-packed with ORS using pouch instructional messages. This design strategy encouraged the use of the product for diarrhea treatment.[144] In Uganda, the switch to co-packaged ORS and zinc played an important role in the increase of both ORS and zinc uptake.[131]

It is paramount for practitioners to evaluate culturally tailored ORS designs, investigate hurdles to community adoption, and address cultural norms. According to a study conducted in Ethiopia, homemade ORS was acceptable as a treatment because of its similarity to a locally prepared cereal, known as buluka (Oromo) or atemeet (Amhara), which enhanced its cultural acceptability.[145]

In the East Shewa Administrative Region of Ethiopia's Adamaboset District, public health experts conducted a randomized field trial to determine the relative efficacy of three ORTs in treating acute childhood diarrhea.[146] Prepackaged glucose and salt solution (GORS), homemade cereal added to a prepackaged salt solution (CBORS), and completely homemade cereal plus salt therapy (CBORS) were the ORTs (CBORT). The study included 463 children under the age of five who had active diarrhea and lived in 18 of the districts. CBORT-using mothers were more likely than CBORS-using mothers, or GORS-using mothers, to follow rehydration therapy directions. CBORT was more culturally acceptable in the community.[146] These findings revealed that homemade ORT has the best potential to reach the greatest number of children, especially in rural communities. Thus, caretakers are more compliant with the treatment if it is made with familiar and culturally accepted ingredients, such as cereal, which improves uptake.

Conclusion

Implementation science can help avoid reinventing the round wheel, which wastes resources. It can also help us reinvent the square wheel, a repetition of learning what does not work in the scale-up of ORS. This continual reinvention costs time, money, and lives. There is evidence and several examples of how implementation science supports the scale-up of ORS in Africa. However, gaps remain. The prospects for closing the remaining ORS delivery gap would increase if implementation research can further inform local applications, preventing reinvention of the wheels by critically examining what works and does not. I would argue that both the bottom-up and top-down approaches can maximize opportunities for accessibility of any ORS for children. Governments can provide policy and guidance instead of having complete control over closing the ORS gap. Implementation science can help discover the nuances that make ORS implementation programs effective or make them failures, particularly in four areas: (1) availability and accessibility, (2) awareness and education among communities, (3) robust partnership engagement strategies, and (4) adaptable design to enhance acceptability.

3
Handwashing and Hygiene: Basic but Crucial

Handwashing with soap has the potential to avert preventable deaths, improve healthcare outcomes, and bolster progress in education, equity, and WASH to achieve the Sustainable Development Goals.

– Global Handwashing Partnership

Africa has a comparatively higher percentage of the population without access to handwashing with soap and water than other areas of the world.[147] In western sub-Saharan Africa, for example, 85.5% of people do not have access to soap and water, which is very high compared with high-income North America at 0.4% or Western Europe at 0.9%.[147]

This chapter explores the historical evolution, present situation, and strategies used to advance handwashing practices in Africa; evaluates the effectiveness and challenges of diverse handwashing initiatives; and outlines critical lessons for improving handwashing in Africa. The quotation that starts this chapter from the Global Handwashing Partnership positions handwashing not just as an individual health measure but also as a powerful tool for achieving the broader goals of the 2030 agenda for sustainable development. It conveys how a basic act like handwashing has transformative potential in enhancing interventions across various sectors, such as nutrition, equity, education, sanitation, and hygiene.

Handwashing compliance is unequal across countries in Africa. A study published in the *Journal of Water, Sanitation and Hygiene for Development* found that the prevalence of a handwashing facility at home was unequal in Kenya, Rwanda, Tanzania, and Uganda, with frequencies of 66.4%, 76.4%, 80.7%, and 59.2%, respectively.[148] The study explained that these differences were associated with the types of interventions in each country.[148] For example, Tanzania effectively used community health extension workers to promote better sanitation practices, whereas the Ugandan government focused more on policy formulation over service delivery.[148] Further, an analysis of Demographic and Health Surveys of 16 countries in sub-Saharan Africa from 2015 to 2018 showed that an average of 33.5% of households had a handwashing area with soap and water, but there was a vast range between countries, with rates of 5% in Burundi and 64% in Angola.[149] Higher wealth and residence in urban settings were associated with having a handwashing area with soap and water.[149]

A systematic review published in 2014 showed that the mean prevalence of handwashing with soap was 14% in Africa compared with 49% in the United States and 52% in the United Kingdom.[150]

Handwashing practice with a disinfecting surfactant agent and water was not known to be an effective method of removing "germs" until 1847, when the aetiology of puerperal sepsis (i.e., an infection of the genital tract postpartum) was discovered by Ignaz Philipp Semmelweis, a Hungarian physician.[151] Semmelweis felt compelled to find the root cause of puerperal sepsis and its contagious transmission when he was appointed as an assistant to Professor Johann Klein in an obstetrical clinic in Vienna, Austria.[152] He witnessed a stark difference between mothers who were attended by medical students and mothers who were attended by midwives. The division with medical students had a death rate of 22.5% from what was then called *childbed fever*, and the midwife division had a 3% mortality rate.[152] This troubled Semmelweis, and he made it his duty to determine the cause by meticulously eliminating possibilities. He even went as far as investigating religious practices. Eventually, he discovered that new infections stemmed from inadequate hand hygiene, transmitting bacteria between medical students and patients.[153]

At that point in the early nineteenth century, miasma theory (i.e., the spread of disease through bad air) was prominent and germ theory had not yet been robustly established by scientists such as Robert Koch and Louis Pasteur. The aetiology of childbed fever was not well understood (it was later known to be streptococcal blood poisoning).[151,152,154] The main difference Semmelweis observed between the two divisions was that medical students were tasked with practising on actual infants in addition to performing other tasks in the hospitals, such as examining patients in the necropsy room. In contrast, midwives primarily worked in the homes of mothers.[152]

Semmelweis hypothesized that particles from cadavers were transferred by the medical students' contaminated hands to patients' genitals and subsequently absorbed into the vascular system.[152] He conducted trials in which he made all staff and students working with patients wash their hands in a chlorinated lime disinfectant, which was reported to have decreased the mortality rate from 12.24% down to 3.04% after 6 months.[155] While this was a groundbreaking discovery, Semmelweis's theory was rejected by the European scientific community because it was perceived to undermine the prestige of the medical profession.[151] Semmelweis's claims went against the conventional wisdom of miasma theory and conflicted with established medical opinion.[153] Semmelweis published his book and research in 1861 on the aetiology of childbed fever.

Florence Nightingale, considered the founder of modern nursing, further pushed the handwashing agenda during the Crimean War (1853–56) in British hospitals to reduce the rates of infections.[151] Nightingale wrote in her nursing book during the Crimea war that nurses' hands ought to be washed frequently because of the unsanitary conditions of war and claimed that her implementation of handwashing practice in British army hospitals reduced mortality rates from 42% to 2%.[156]

However, despite both Semmelweis's and Nightingale's efforts to persuade the European scientific community of the importance of handwashing and to promote handwashing behaviours, handwashing was not widely adopted until the 1980s.[151] Semmelweis had difficulty providing a scientific basis and acceptable explanation for his claims on handwashing, as the germ theory of disease had not yet been developed to support his findings.[153]

The Emergence of Hand Hygiene for Population Health

It was not until 1981 that the CDC published the first international guideline on preventing and controlling healthcare-associated infections in hospitals with proper hand hygiene. After that, the adoption of handwashing practices increased.[157]

In 1985 the CDC published its most notable and first highly influential record of handwashing.[158] The official hand hygiene guideline was a milestone in public acceptance of the concept of hand hygiene in healthcare; many countries began to follow this guideline after its publication.[151] This document highlighted the connection between poor hand hygiene and healthcare-associated infections, in which a healthcare worker's hands are the most common vehicle for pathogen transmission.[151]

The first iteration of the CDC guideline in 1981 recommended washing hands with plain soap or antimicrobial handwashing products before and after invasive procedures and when taking care of susceptible patients.[158] Two more iterations followed with additional guidelines: the 1995 version added instructions for surgical hand preparation, skin care, and fingernails, and the 2002 version stressed education, motivation, and administration as major factors in prioritizing hand hygiene compliance.[157]

As the 2002 iteration of the CDC guideline stated, a multidisciplinary approach was required to improve hand hygiene compliance in hospital settings.[157] Accountable partners should have been medical institutions (e.g., hospitals, health clinics), educational institutions (e.g., medical schools, nursing schools), and governments. However, this was not necessarily the case.

One study reviewed data from 40 American hospitals in the National Nosocomial Infections Surveillance System and found that although the hospitals changed their policies and procedures to comply with the CDC's guidelines, there was no evidence of actual change in handwashing practice.[157] Long-lasting adoption of new changes to clinical practice guidelines requires a collaborative effort that depends on the support and commitment of the critical parties.[159]

The prevalence and recognition of handwashing on a global scale was further pushed by the Save Lives: Clean Your Hands Initiative that accompanied the WHO's *Guidelines on Hand Hygiene in Health Care* in 2009.[160,161] While convergent with the CDC guideline, the WHO guideline also provided "a comprehensive overview of essential aspects of hand hygiene in health care and evidence- and consensus-based recommendations" and lessons learned from testing implementation tools.[160(p.4)]

Literature on handwashing guidelines has been historically prevalent in European and Western contexts. In 1899, the Liverpool School of Tropical Medicine facilitated an expedition to Freetown to identify mosquito breeding pools, as malaria was prevalent. In 2000, the United Nations Millennium Declaration was signed that committed world leaders to eradicating world poverty, hunger, disease, illiteracy, environmental degradation, and discrimination against women with a target date of the year 2015.[162] These commitments were structured into eight Millennium Development Goals (MDGs), which targeted improved sanitation and hygiene in countries around the world (including those in Africa) that alluded to improving handwashing practices.[162]

Before 2000, the importance placed on handwashing was mixed. In 1994, West Africa experienced a cholera outbreak, but funeral workers and the villagers of Biombo, Guinea-Bissau, rarely used soap for handwashing.[163] Conversely, in 1985, a hospital in a refugee camp in eastern Sudan highly encouraged handwashing, and hospital staff chlorinated water tanks specifically for handwashing.[164] In 1996, two researchers from Johns Hopkins University published a technical paper on the control of epidemic dysentery in Africa. It outlined the absence of soap in the household and the lack of soap use as a risk factor for infectious disease in many African countries such as Burundi and Zambia.[165]

The MDGs were superseded by the Sustainability Development Goals (SDGs), a new roster of 17 goals, and handwashing with soap was explicitly mentioned in SDG 6 for "ensuring availability and sustainable management of water and sanitation for all."[166] Since the uptick in handwashing advocacy, the Global Handwashing Day (held every year on October 15) was launched in 2008 by an international committee of private sector entities, academic institutions, multilateral and governmental agencies, and non-governmental and community-led organizations.[167]

Taking Handwashing Practice to Scale in Clinical Settings

In the COVID-19 pandemic, handwashing became an effective infection control mechanism and preventative measure against contracting SARS-CoV2.[168] However, low compliance in handwashing is still a significant challenge, even in clinical settings. For example, a review of 96 empirical studies revealed a hand hygiene compliance rate in intensive care units of 30% to 40%. Potential factors associated with compliance behaviour include profession, workload, attitude, time of day, patient's risk of infection, feedback, knowledge, and the accessibility of materials.[169]

Global programs have tried to improve handwashing/hand hygiene in clinical settings. For example, the Global Handwashing Partnership is a coalition that brings together resources from private and public sectors around the globe to promote handwashing with soap.[170] For instance, the Partnership uses social media to promote Global Handwashing Day, advocate for handwashing, and encourage people to find creative ways to wash their hands with soap.

The Hand Hygiene for All global initiative was implemented by the WHO to provide recommendations on hand hygiene to control the COVID-19 pandemic.[171] Alongside UNICEF, it called on countries to bridge national COVID-19 preparedness and response plans with mid- and long-term national development plans to ensure proper hand hygiene throughout the pandemic. This also improves infection prevention and control, as well as water, sanitation, and hygiene efforts. The initiative's three major steps are responding to the immediate pandemic, rebuilding infrastructure and services, and reimagining hand hygiene in society.[171]

The World Bank has also funded several seminal handwashing projects around the world, such as the Community Based Drinking Water Supply and Sanitation Program in Indonesia. This project uses a community-based approach to promote behaviour change for the adoption of good hygiene behaviours and practices, such as implementing hand hygiene programs.[172] As reported in a results briefing, this program reached well beyond its target, with 68% of the target communities adopting handwashing programs.[173]

Since 2017, the World Bank has funded the Sustainable Rural Water Supply and Sanitation Project in Kyrgyz Republic in Central Asia. This project targets homes and schools in rural communities to "increase access to improved water and sanitation services" by promoting good hygiene practices such as handwashing.[172]

In Kenya, a hospital-based hand hygiene improvement program involved training staff members at three different hospitals to produce an alcohol-based hand rub.[174] Focus group discussions took place to evaluate its use and found it helped raise hand hygiene compliance from 28% to 38%.

UNICEF and the WHO have also developed the Water, Sanitation, and Hygiene (WASH) program to improve healthcare. They developed eight steps to improve WASH in healthcare facilities: conducting condition situation analysis and assessment, setting targets and defining road maps, establishing national standards and accountability mechanisms, improving and maintaining infrastructure, monitoring and reviewing the data, developing the health workforce, engaging communities, and conducting operational research and sharing learning.[175]

The Turn Africa Orange program initiative by the Infection Control Africa Network[176] encouraged African countries to participate in enlisting healthcare facilities to improve hand hygiene. The phrase *turn orange* referred to the African countries that were mapped by the number of healthcare facilities registered with the Save Lives: Clean Your Hands campaign by the WHO. The colours from red to pale yellow referred to the density of the number of healthcare facilities, and the goal was to move from yellow (few) to orange (many).[176] The program used multi-modal strategies and methodological tools from the WHO to implement hand hygiene programs, such as raising awareness of healthcare-associated infections, improving organization of healthcare delivery, and acquiring new effective attitudes that place importance on teamwork.[176]

The Aurum Institute, a health impact organization and implementing partner for the CDC in South Africa, launched innovative mobile hand hygiene stations called Shesha Geza, which translates to "hurry up and wash" in isiZulu.[177] These stations were allocated to public health facilities across the Ekurhuleni in the Gauteng Province to combat COVID-19.[177] Fifteen stations were distributed in phase one at a cost of ZAR 375,000 (USD 28,397) and another 36 stations in phase two.[178] The stations can provide over 20,000 handwashes before needing a refill.[178]

In particular, this innovation was funded by the CDC South Africa.[178] It was developed by Aurum Innova, a division of the Aurum Institute. Aurum Innova is a digital healthcare innovation company that focuses on social enterprise to impact grassroots communities and provides expertise to the South African government, the private sector, and civil society.[179] Because the innovation started in a grassroots community level, a key lesson from Shesha Geza is that drawing from local inspiration and creativity contributes to the successful creation of partnerships.[178]

Taking Handwashing Practice to Scale in Community Settings

Several innovative programs, such as the Tippy Tap challenge by UNICEF, encouraged young people to engage in the COVID-19 response. A Tippy Tap is a simple handwashing mechanism that uses little water, a plastic bottle, string, sticks, and soap for convenient and practical handwashing based on limited resources. For each one they build, young people earn digital rewards that can be redeemed for food or airline vouchers through UNICEF's partnership with Zlto. Zlto counts it as a work asset that young people can use when applying for a job.[180]

In South Africa, 72 handwashing stations funded by Woolworths and its partnership with UNICEF have been made for schools, available for students and faculty to use to improve handwashing compliance.[53] Handwashing rates in South Africa are currently low, mainly in rural populations, with Madagascar, Lesotho, Zimbabwe, Zambia, and Swaziland having a handwashing rate of less than 25% in rural areas.[181]

In West Africa, we see a great example in Ghana. The Greater Accra Metropolitan Area Sanitation and Water Project for Ghana is a grant of USD 150 million given by the World Bank to the Government of Ghana to increase access to sanitation and a water supply.[182] The main objectives of the project are to provide environmental sanitation and water supply services to low-income areas, to improve and expand the water distribution network, and to strengthen institutions in sanitation management.[182] Included in these objectives is the improvement of handwashing facilities.[172]

Community-led total sanitation (CLTS) has been implemented in at least 18 countries in Africa. CLTS is a methodology created by Kamal Kar, a development consultant from India, and the Village Education Research Center, a partner of WaterAid Bangladesh.[183] Historically, CLTS was created in Mosmoil, a village in Bangladesh, when Kar was evaluating its subsidized sanitation program.[183] He realized that he needed to persuade the Village Education Research Center to change its traditional sanitation program's approach and advocate for having villagers analyze their waste situation and make communal collective decisions to end open defecation.[183] CLTS focuses on behaviour change in communities to stop open defecation by using behavioural and psychological triggers.

Included in this comprehensive approach is the trigger to wash hands at key events after defecation.[183] The CLTS approach has been implemented in several countries, including Angola, Botswana, Burundi, Djibouti, Eritrea, Ethiopia, Kenya, Madagascar, Malawi, Mozambique, Namibia, Somalia, South Africa, South Sudan, Sudan, Tanzania, Uganda, Zambia, and Zimbabwe.[183]

In terms of impact, a mixed-methods systematic review in 2018 concluded that the evidence of CLTS's effectiveness is weak and that more rigorous research on CLTS is required.[184] However, another study evaluated the outcomes of four CLTS programs in Ethiopia and Ghana, concluding that CLTS outcomes can be sustained with trained local actors and that program applicability is dependent on local context.[185] Finally, a report on CLTS implementation in Busia, Kenya, stated the importance of local context; community leaders promoting CLTS in rural communities socially has an impact on CLTS adoption in those communities.[186]

Handwashing Programs in Africa

Tippy Tap Technology

One systematic review investigated the use of Tippy Taps in resource-limited settings and found that the availability of Tippy Taps increased the frequency of handwashing with soap and water.[187] Seventeen of the 20 studies that were reviewed took place in African countries.[187] The Tippy Tap is affordable because of the inexpensive materials required for construction, often just a small jerrycan, a wooden frame, and some string.[187] The low cost of the Tippy Tap made it easy and accessible for many households to construct one on their own.[187] According to a case study of Tippy Taps in Uganda, a number of implications arose when it came to scaling up. The dissemination of Tippy Tap knowledge was limited between and within villages because of isolation.[188] Furthermore, the distribution of Tippy Taps was labour-intensive and relied on village health team volunteers, who were limited by time and physical reach.[188] A lesson that can be drawn from these studies is that the low cost and availability of supplies and resources can create an intervention; however, that alone is not enough to achieve handwashing goals. A comprehensive strategy is required in which the social environment must also be able to foster the adoption of Tippy Taps.

To illustrate, a school in rural Uganda implemented a handwashing program that used Tippy Taps and had an improved handwashing rate one month after implementation.[189] This program was successful because the school children were actively participating in the health learning process by constructing the Tippy Taps, they enjoyed washing their hands with Tippy Taps specifically, and they told their families at home what they had learned about handwashing.[189] These outcomes were also largely dependent on the availability of cost-effective materials: one Tippy Tap costs USD 2 to make, and its maintenance costs USD 0.06 per student per month.[189]

Social Art for Behaviour Change

WaterAid, an international NGO for WASH, collaborated with the One Drop Foundation, another NGO for WASH, in Mali in 2017. An approach called the Social Art for Behaviour Change, whose purpose is to inspire, activate, and sustain behaviour change through social and artistic modalities, was used in the villages of Mali to drive behaviour change towards sustained handwashing practices.[190] This was done in produced shows about themes related to handwashing practices, radio programs, short films, and paintings.[191] In particular, this approach is part of a larger model, called the ABC for Sustainability model, consisting of three elements: safe and equitable access to services, behaviour change through social art interventions, and capital for supporting market-based solutions.[190] As part of a larger model and initiative, the Social Art for Behaviour Change approach has improved the living conditions of over 2.7 million people worldwide, and 721,595 people in Africa specifically, as of December 2022.[192] A lesson on implementation that other initiatives can use is to incorporate an artistic process, creativity, and co-creation elements in an intervention to inspire behaviour change (e.g., handwashing behaviour) on an emotional level. For example, creating a mural was an initiative in Guatemala and Sweden, where community members painted their handprints onto a mural representing ownership and involvement in improving WASH behaviours.[193]

Homemade Soapy Water System

The economic driver of the affordability of handwash materials was also identified in a study done in Bangladesh. This study followed a health promotion program that distributed a "soapy water system," which consisted of a 1.5 L plastic water bottle that dispensed a mixture of water and detergent that cost USD 0.03 per 1.5 L.[194] The study reported that households accepted this technology as it was cheap to sustain and easy to share with other unrelated families.[194] For example, this study specifically focused on households in low-income neighbourhoods, in which the intervention implemented was a combination of the provision of soapy water bottles and the educational element of community health promoters who conduct courtyard meetings with community members.[194] Similar to lessons noted above, social elements need to be factored in for implementation success; the inclusion of community lead roles (e.g., landlords, compound managers) could improve community engagement and strengthen the sense of leadership in compounds that need additional support in a shared soapy water system.[194]

Similar to a soapy water system, soap alternative technologies such as the Povu Poa model developed in Kenya are cost-effective and are strong facilitators of handwashing in resource-constrained settings.[195] This technology consists of a water reservoir (e.g., bucket, pipe) with a frugal water tap and a soap-foaming dispenser that costs USD 0.10 for 100 handwashes.[195] A complete unit costs an estimated USD 12 for mass production and deployment.[195]

Handwashing Implementation Lessons for Africa

A systematic review across 46 articles published between 2003 and 2020 uncovered vital challenges and facilitators to handwashing.[196] The critical factors to scaling up the practice of handwashing revolved around seven broad vital areas: (1) champions, (2) cost and affordability, (3) funding and resources, (4) sustainability and capabilities, (5) time management, (6) gender and adaptability, and (7) health promotion. These identified themes provide a framework for developing strategies to strengthen community handwashing with soap and water.

Champions: Individual compliance in handwashing practices can be influenced significantly by a role model or champion.[197,198] In a refugee camp in Northern Kenya, a three-year-old girl named Farhiya was a champion as she demonstrated to the other children in the camp how to wash their hands. According to Farhiya, she was taught how to wash her hands by her father, a Catholic Relief Services employee, to remove dirt and germs that could make her ill. Farhiya probably preserved the lives of a few of her friends, because hundreds of thousands of Somali refugees like her were crowded into the camp, and disease spread quickly. Though Farhiya may not have been aware of the precise link between germs and diarrhea, she had mastered the act of washing hands thoroughly and she was a champion. Dig Deep (a non-profit organization) has invested in WASH champions who have been trained as Trainers of Trainers. School teachers and community health volunteers are trained as WASH champions, and then they educate their peers, students, and children about good hygiene practices (including thorough handwashing with soap).

Cost: One of the main recommendations made by the WHO to control the COVID-19 pandemic was frequent handwashing; nevertheless, the cost of having adequate handwashing facilities was a major obstacle to preventing the spread of infection in regions lacking a reliable and clean water supply. An affordable, simple, and efficient handwashing technology was required to encourage people to wash their hands. As discussed above, the Tippy Tap challenge initiative was then developed in South Africa by UNICEF to curb the spread of COVID-19 and prevent a comeback by constructing simple and low-cost handwashing facilities, particularly in high-risk communities. During the Tippy Tap challenge, the students in Limekhaya Secondary School also constructed a handwashing station inside the school.[199] According to Naughton et al.,[200] Tippy Tap may be exactly what is needed to successfully adopt handwashing behaviour because the stations are easily constructed, affordable, and made of local materials.

Funding and resources: One of the primary barriers to effective handwashing practice is a lack of resources or inadequate funds to purchase enough resources for effective handwashing. For example, soap, a required resource for effective handwashing, was lacking in refugee camps in Kenya and Ethiopia.[201] The few soaps available were prioritized for laundry and bathing above handwashing. When refugees did wash their hands, it was because free soap was widely available in the camp. Therefore, increasing the availability of soap will be useful in improving safe handwashing practices.[201] The people living in the Soweto slum of Nairobi couldn't afford to buy soap to wash their hands. To increase handwashing, a charity organization called the Tulid Child Trust developed and distributed vegetable-based soap.[202]

Sustainability and capability: The term *sustainability* refers to the extent to which an intervention can deliver its intended benefits over an extended period.[203] Holmen et al.[204] argued that it is challenging to achieve the long-term sustainability of handwashing interventions in low-income settings, particularly in rural low-income areas. Lack of access to water and soap in Kenyan schools contributes significantly to the low prevalence of handwashing. Several interventions and efforts have been made to promote handwashing in schools.[205] Some of these efforts included budgeting for soap purchases to overcome the lack of soap, employing a WASH attendant to ensure the availability of water and soap, and substituting an alcohol-based hand sanitizer for bar soap.[206,207] However, the cost of sustaining these efforts was high. As a result, Povu Poa, a longer-lasting intervention, was designed and developed. The Povu Poa is a portable handwashing system that uses a water-saving tap and a cost-effective soap foam dispenser.[205] The Povu Poa comes in a bucket stand model and a pipe model, and it is designed to save water and soap use while promoting the hygienic aspects of handwashing.[205] Tippy Tap, the handwashing facility in Mali, is stationed outside in the open compound. Unfortunately, many families keep goats, sheep, and cows, which eat and destroy the soap and damage the handwashing stations when people are sleeping or working in the fields. To sustain this technology, a sardine can was added to the Tippy Tap design to protect the soap from damage, and the wooden foot pedal was replaced with bamboo as a more durable material.[200]

Time management: Time is one of the crucial factors that influence handwashing behaviours. Lack of time has been reported as a reason that pupils and teachers may not wash their hands properly or at all.[208] Also, according to a study done among Kenyan students, the experience of waiting in long lines for handwashing was a major factor that discouraged handwashing behaviours among students.[209]

Gender and adaptability: Mothers have a crucial role in children's health behaviour because they are the children's closest and most dependable caregivers. During the COVID-19 pandemic, mothers in Juba (Juba is the capital and largest city of South Sudan) were educated on the importance of handwashing and hygiene practice. Fortunately, after gaining knowledge of the value of handwashing, mothers in Juba started to practise handwashing and hygiene to protect their families from COVID-19. For instance, Merlin Benson, a mother to 9-month-old Sarah, stated that "this disease is so terrifying. I will make sure my baby and I are safe by following the advice shared at the nutrition centre." Also, Jackeline Albino, a mother of four, said that she "visited the hospital twice monthly due to frequent diarrhea and infection. After learning and practicing handwashing with clean water to prevent diseases, she is healthier. Now, she makes sure her children's hands are washed before and after eating and going to the toilet."[210]

Health promotion: Handwashing promotion programs aim to increase knowledge and influence handwashing behaviour. For instance, four primary schools in Tanzania participated in the Mikono Safi health promotion program, which included soap and water demonstrations to teach kids about appropriate hand cleanliness. The Mikono Safi (Kiswahili for "clean hands") intervention was designed to increase handwashing with soap among school-age children.[211] An assessment of the Mikono Safi program indicated that the program boosted students' capability and motivation to wash their hands with soap at critical times, particularly after using the toilet. Improvements in students' handwashing knowledge and skills were reported by both teachers and students, and emotional drivers like disgust, fear, and nurture increased motivation for handwashing.[211] During the Ebola pandemic in the Democratic Republic of the Congo, the WHO and other partner organizations helped the government combat the epidemic by funding campaigns and health programs that promoted handwashing and other hygienic practices. Children from Katsya School in the Democratic Republic of the Congo participated in one of the health promotion programs to instil the importance of hand hygiene. Through song and dance, the children of Katsya School learned how good hand hygiene could help protect their health and their families from Ebola. The children were urged to model good handwashing behaviour at home.

Conclusion

Effective approaches to improving handwashing play a crucial role in enhancing hygiene practices. Grassroots innovations, local partnerships, and affordable technologies can effectively improve hand hygiene. A comprehensive approach is essential, addressing not only the technical aspects of handwashing but also the social and behavioural factors that influence adoption. Key lessons include the need for sustained funding, community engagement, and adaptable solutions to ensure long-term success in promoting handwashing behaviours and reducing disease transmission in resource-constrained settings.

4
Neglected Tropical Diseases Innovations: The Forgotten

The most shocking aspect of NTDs isn't the devastation they can cause to poor communities; it's the affordability of its solution.

– Dr. Peter Hotez

On 15 February 2022, I listened to WHO directors and advisers discuss the launch of the WHO guideline on the control and elimination of human schistosomiasis as a public health problem. Three things occurred to me as I watched the webinar. First, the progress that has been made in the treatment and prevention of neglected tropical diseases (NTDs) over the last 30 years has been impressive; second, the importance of WASH as a critical element of schistosomiasis control and treatment has been recognized; and finally, the radical transformation of schistosomiasis control became possible through a very affordable innovation, a drug created more than 50 years ago – praziquantel.

This chapter delves into the history and development of praziquantel, examines several critical initiatives in the scale-up of the mass drug administration (MDA) of praziquantel, and investigates some lessons learned in implementing MDA over the last several decades. The quotation at the beginning of the chapter from Dr. Peter Hotez, published on the HuffPost Contributor platform in 2012, uncovers a paradox: while NTDs such as schistosomiasis overwhelm the world's poorest populations, the means to prevent and treat them, such as praziquantel, are surprisingly cost-effective.[212]

Praziquantel was developed in the 1970s by the German pharmaceutical firms Bayer A.G., now known as Bayer Schering Pharma, and E. Merck, now known as Merck KGaA.[213] Tranquillizers were assessed to treat the parasitic and prevalent disease schistosomiasis, with minimal side effects, leading to the pyrazinoisoquinoline group being tested; however, high doses were required for it to be as effective as known tranquillizers. The compounds in this group then went on for veterinary screening.[214] From 400 compounds, praziquantel was selected and was found to be an effective anthelminthic against various parasites and cestodes.[213]

In December 1973, praziquantel was patented in Germany as a veterinary anthelminthic and then in 1977 in the United States.[215] Bayer and Merck registered the patent for praziquantel in 38 countries. In the late 1970s, Bayer also worked with the WHO to conduct clinical trials for praziquantel's safety in humans.[215]

Found successful against many platyhelminths in humans, praziquantel began its spread worldwide.[215] Praziquantel became available in Europe after 1978 and on the international market in the 1980s.[216] It was seen as the main drug of choice against schistosomiasis because of its efficacy, low toxicity, and ease of single oral dose.[217,218] One dose of praziquantel (40 mg/kg body weight) was known to treat schistosomiasis but not prevent it, and by 1984 about 1 million people had been treated.[218]

In the early 1980s, South Korean firm Shin Poong Pharmaceutical Co saw how praziquantel could treat schistosomiasis and liver fluke.[215] Wanting to make it more accessible internationally, Shin Poong created an alternative cost-effective process for producing praziquantel and received a government-protected patent to do so. This new production reduced schistosomiasis in Korea from 41% in 1981 to 4% in 1983 and liver fluke from 2.6% in 1981 to 2.2% in 1993.[215]

In the early 1990s, Shin Poong was the world's largest producer of praziquantel. As part of the international production strategy, Shin Poong registered the new product and received a patent to produce it in 12 other countries and licensing arrangements in other countries.[215] The 12 countries were Bangladesh, Germany, India, Italy, Japan, Pakistan, Peru, Taiwan, Thailand, United Kingdom, United States of America, and Venezuela.[215] Shin Poong exported large volumes of praziquantel to several European and African countries, such as Malawi, Sudan, Uganda, Switzerland, Ghana, Tanzania, and Zimbabwe.[215]

In Egypt, the Egyptian International Pharmaceutical Industries Co. began manufacturing praziquantel in 1987 under a licensing agreement with Shin Poong.[215] Then, starting in 1988, the Ministry of Health in Egypt provided praziquantel for free as part of their national schistosomiasis control program.[215] Praziquantel was given to infected persons based on diagnosis, which significantly reduced the prevalence of schistosomiasis in numerous studies, showing similar efficacy nationally.[219,220] In

1993, Egypt sold 10 million tablets of praziquantel annually, with about 2 million more tablet sales in the private market.[215]

Today, praziquantel is being scaled up in Africa through various means, including providing free praziquantel treatment to school-age children (SAC), ages 5 to 14, as well as adults, who live in disease endemic areas.[221,222] In 2001, the World Health Assembly aimed to treat 75% of SAC globally by 2010.[223] In 2012 the WHO created a road map to assist with scale-up strategies to ensure increased accessibility and treatment with praziquantel.[223]

In 2021 the WHO published its road map for NTDs from 2021 to 2030, which highlighted the need to innovate and scale up diagnostic tests, detect resistance to praziquantel, find alternative medication, ensure access to praziquantel through donations (250 million tablets of praziquantel from Merck for African communities and children), and treat at-risk groups (SAC and preschool-age children, communities in high endemic locations, and adults in occupations with contact with unclean water). [224] Praziquantel is the main chemotherapeutic drug of choice because of its effectiveness against all schistosome species, its affordability, and its safety compared with other chemotherapeutic drugs.[225] A drawback, however, is that the large tablets and bitter taste make it less suitable for children who often need it the most.[226]

Praziquantel MDA in Africa

Before the early 2000s, preventive chemotherapy with praziquantel was not widely used in sub-Saharan Africa; however, this changed in 2005 when Merck pledged to provide 250 million praziquantel tablets yearly.[223] From 2002 onwards, preventive chemotherapy efforts for schistosomiasis were scaled up in the form of MDA programs. According to a WHO report, praziquantel was administered to roughly 762 million SAC and 191 million adults in 2018, resulting in 61.2% treatment coverage for children and 18.2% treatment coverage for adults, in contrast to 2006, when only 7 million people were treated.[227]

Despite significant progress in recent years in African countries to consistently implement MDA of praziquantel, the national achievement remains far short of the WHO's target of regular MDA to at least 75% of SAC at risk.[228] In 2015, only nine countries reached that WHO target threshold for the treatment of at least 75% of SAC in the African region.[229] However, in 2017, the number increased to 17 of the 40 African countries in which treatment is required.[227] Therefore, there is still a need to strengthen program performance to scale up the MDA of praziquantel and increase the coverage in African countries.

The WHO has made significant efforts over the last 20 years to scale up the MDA of praziquantel in Africa. In 2001, the World Health Assembly passed the WHA54.19 resolution, emphasizing morbidity control through preventive chemotherapy with praziquantel as the global strategy. As noted, the target for MDA was at least 75% and up to 100% of SAC by 2010.[230] This resolution generated a greater political commitment in many member states.[230] Following this resolution, great progress has been made in scaling up the MDA of praziquantel in Africa. This was accomplished as a result of the favourable response of international organizations and NGOs to the WHO's 2001 call to action.[231] Millions of children are regularly treated with praziquantel, thanks to USAID, the UK DFID, the Bill and Melinda Gates Foundation, the pharmaceutical sector, and various non-profit organizations.[231]

In January 2012 the WHO released a road map for NTDs that set targets for 2012 to 2020. The road map outlined the strategic approach to scale up preventive chemotherapy treatment for schistosomiasis.[231] Partners (pharmaceutical industries, donors, and NGOs) also accepted the London declaration on NTDs, pledging to support the WHO road map and its 10 NTD targets by 2020.[231] Also in 2012, the World Health Assembly passed a resolution on the elimination of schistosomiasis by WHO member states.[231] The resolution urged all epidemic countries, particularly those in Africa, to scale up control interventions, strengthen surveillance, and ensure access to praziquantel.[231] The resolution garnered overwhelming support from the pharmaceutical industry, which led to the donation of praziquantel.[231] The resolution calls for continuous country ownership of NTD prevention programs. African governments were urged to take responsibility for increasing schistosomiasis treatment coverage in their countries. The WHO recommends that African countries should source funding to implement MDA and also devise a unique strategy to achieve and maintain universal access to and coverage of praziquantel.[231] As of 2016, 36 African countries had established and launched their national master plans for NTD control, which included measures for increasing the MDA of praziquantel for schistosomiasis.[222]

The WHO Regional Office for Africa (AFRO) initiated a mapping program in January 2014 with the goal of completing schistosomiasis mapping in all African countries.[228] Even though African countries have a disproportionately high burden of schistosomiasis, the mapping of disease prevalence in many of them remains incomplete. This initiative, funded by the Bill and Melinda Gates Foundation, accelerated the completion of schistosomiasis mapping in the WHO African region. By June 2016, prevalence mapping for schistosomiasis had been completed in 41 of the 47 WHO African regions,[232] and millions of children are regularly treated with praziquantel.

Nine years after the WHO released its first road map for NTDs, the MDA of praziquantel was successfully scaled to a significant level thanks to exceptional leadership and continued support from pharmaceutical industries and international organizations. However, several African nations failed to meet the WHO target for MDA coverage. In 2020, another road map for NTDs for 2021 to 2030 was developed by the WHO through extensive global consultation of the executive board. This new road map was based on previous lessons and experiences, and it identified critical gaps and measures needed to meet the 2030 schistosomiasis elimination and control aim.[228] The road map aims to eliminate schistosomiasis as a public health issue by 2030, as well as to stop schistosome transmission in humans in selected nations. Preventive treatment of at-risk people is one of the key strategies recommended by the WHO for controlling and eliminating human schistosomiasis.[228] The major critical action for 2021–30 set by the WHO is to expand preventive chemotherapy (praziquantel) to all populations in need and to ensure access to praziquantel in African countries.[228]

As part of the World Neglected Tropical Diseases Day 2022 celebrations, the WHO released a new guideline for the control and elimination of schistosomiasis. The guidelines provide African countries with evidence-based recommendations for controlling and eliminating schistosomiasis as a public health problem.[228] The expansion of preventive chemotherapy eligibility from the predominant group of SAC to all age groups, including preschool-age children and adults, and the emphasis on lowering the prevalence threshold for annual preventive chemotherapy are the key stand-out recommendations in this new guideline.[228] These are the first schistosomiasis guidelines approved by the WHO guideline review committee. The previous implementation guidelines for schistosomiasis were primarily based on expert opinion.[228] However, this new guideline provides evidence-based recommendations. There was no previously published guidance on the evaluation of schistosomiasis transmission interruption.[228] These recommendations will be useful for African countries in scaling up national schistosomiasis and elimination programs, such as the praziquantel MDA. The guideline urges countries to expand and ensure consistency of preventive chemotherapy programs.[228] The WHO recommends annual preventive chemotherapy with a single dose of praziquantel at 75% treatment coverage in all age groups from 2 years old, including adults, pregnant women after the first trimester, and lactating women.[228]

Over the years, there has been a considerable increase in the scale-up of MDA of praziquantel in Africa, thanks to the commitment and support of WHO partners. Merck KGaA committed to increasing the supply of praziquantel to reach 250 million tablets per year, which is equivalent to 100 million treatments for SAC.[228] Through the WHO, the donated praziquantel tablets are being delivered to endemic African countries such as Nigeria, Sudan, and Ethiopia. Other donors, such as the USAID, the UK DFID (now Foreign, Commonwealth and Development Office), and World Vision, were committed to providing both praziquantel for treatment and funding for implementation of MDA in several African countries. In 2004, with the support of the Bill and Melinda Gates Foundation through the Schistosomiasis Control Initiative, national control programs were launched in Burkina Faso, Mali, and Niger.[233]

Critical Initiatives in the Scale-Up of Praziquantel MDA in Africa

Schistosomiasis is most common in tropical and subtropical regions, especially among impoverished people lacking access to safe drinking water and adequate sanitation.[234] Africa accounts for approximately 93% of the world's schistosomiasis cases, with the highest prevalence reported in Nigeria, Malawi, Uganda, Tanzania, Ghana, Mozambique, and the Democratic Republic of the Congo.[235]

A report from the WHO revealed that about 90% of those requiring treatment for schistosomiasis live in Africa.[228] In Africa, there has been a significant increase in the mass treatment of schistosomiasis over the years. For instance, in 2010, about 57 million Nigerians required preventive chemotherapy treatment. Sadly, only about 2.3 million received treatment.[234] By 2020, out of the 26 million Nigerians that required praziquantel, about 16 million were treated.[234] Also, in Uganda, in 2014, about 10.4 million of the population required treatment for schistosomiasis; only 2.7 million were treated. By 2020, 12.3 million of Ugandans required praziquantel, and about 5.3 million were treated.[234]

The low availability of praziquantel, either for purchase or donation, posed a significant challenge to the scale-up of preventative chemotherapy in sub-Saharan Africa to control schistosomiasis.[236] With the expansion of the Schistosomiasis Control Initiative's efforts beginning in 2002, it was evident that the future demand for significant quantities of praziquantel would increase.[237] In collaboration with the WHO, Merck KGaA, a leading scientific and technology business, has provided 1.5 billion praziquantel tablets.[238] Since 2007, Merck has facilitated the distribution of praziquantel to around 600 million SAC in 47 sub-Saharan

Figure 4.1. Prevalence of Schistosomiasis in the WHO African Region

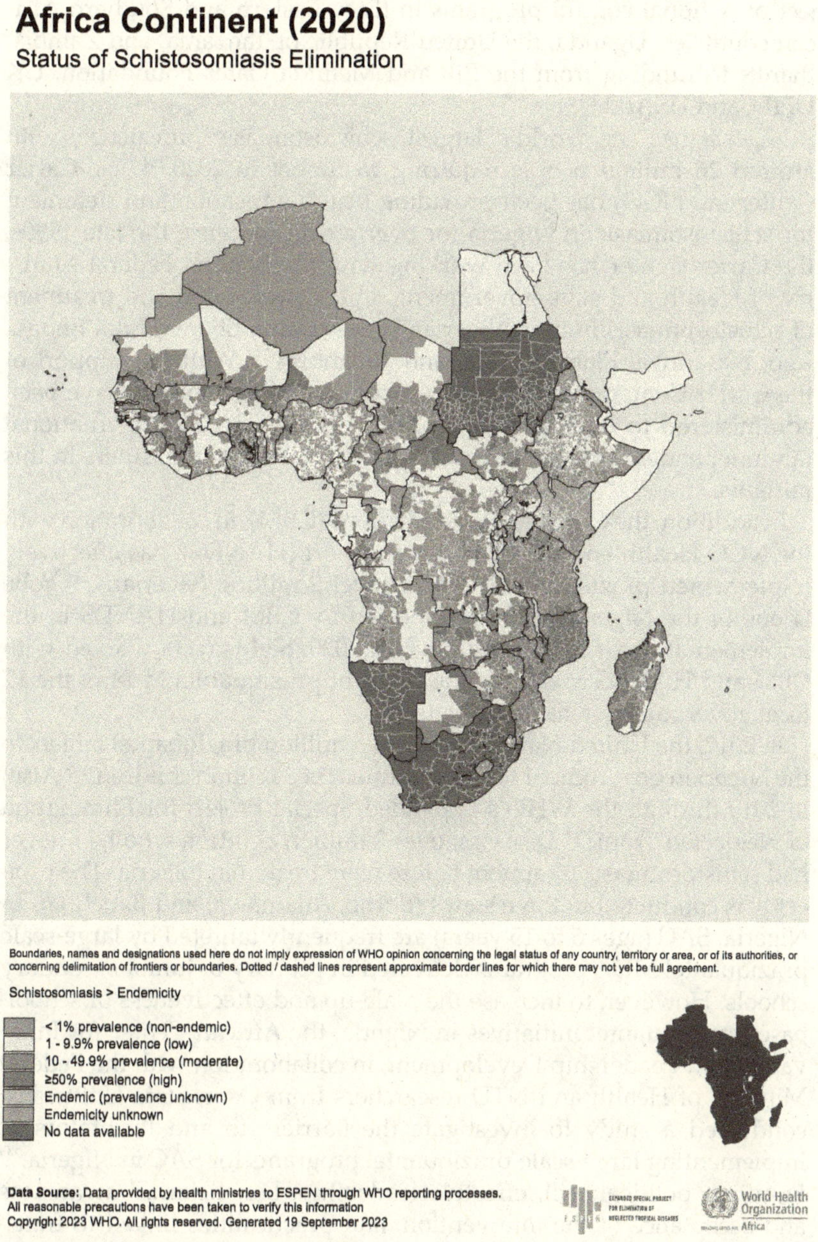

Africa Continent (2020)

Status of Schistosomiasis Elimination

Boundaries, names and designations used here do not imply expression of WHO opinion concerning the legal status of any country, territory or area, or of its authorities, or concerning delimitation of frontiers or boundaries. Dotted / dashed lines represent approximate border lines for which there may not yet be full agreement.

Schistosomiasis > Endemicity

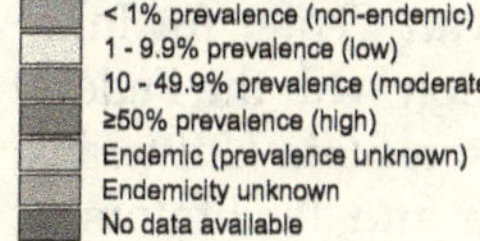

Data Source: Data provided by health ministries to ESPEN through WHO reporting processes.
All reasonable precautions have been taken to verify this information

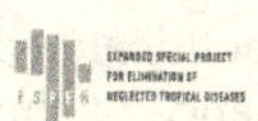

Source: Status of Schistosomiasis Elimination. African Region (AFRO): World Health Organization; 2020. Licence: CC BY-NC-SA 3.0 IGO.

African and other nations.[238] Schistosomiasis control has been the subject of national control programs in three Eastern and Southern African countries: Uganda, the United Republic of Tanzania, and Zambia, thanks to funding from the Bill and Melinda Gates Foundation, UK DFID, and USAID.[239]

Nigeria has the world's largest schistosomiasis prevalence, with around 26 million people requiring treatment in 2020.[234] The Carter Center (an NGO) has been providing health education and treatment for schistosomiasis in Nigeria for over a decade. Since the late 1990s, the Carter Center has been working with the Nigeria Federal Ministry of Health and state governments in the prevention and treatment of schistosomiasis in nine Nigerian states (Delta, Ebonyi, Edo, Enugu, Imo, Nasarawa, Plateau, Abia, and Anambra).[240] With the support of the Carter Center, over 28 million praziquantel treatments have been administered to Nigerians since 1999. USAID and RTI International (an independent non-profit research institute) are key partners in this initiative.[240]

In addition, the Christian Blind Missions (CBM), in collaboration with the NGO Health and Development Support (HANDS), has effectively implemented praziquantel MDA for over 2 million Nigerians.[241] Yobe is one of the Nigerian states supported by CBM and HANDS in the implementation of NTD programs. In 2020, Sightsavers worked with CBM and HANDS to deliver the MDA of praziquantel in 14 of the 17 local government areas in the state.[242]

In 2012, the United Nations donated 5 million praziquantel tablets to the Nigerian government for the treatment of 3 million children.[243] Also, in 2019 through the WHO's Expanded Special Project for Elimination of Neglected Tropical Diseases, over 2 million children who had never had schistosomiasis treatment before were treated in Nigeria. The project was conducted in three states (Borno, Adamawa, and Bauchi).[227] In Nigeria, SAC (ages 6 to 15 years) are frequently targeted by large-scale praziquantel MDA programs delivered in primary or junior secondary schools. However, to increase the scale-up and effectiveness of school-based praziquantel initiatives in Nigeria, the African Center for Innovation and Leadership Development, in collaboration with the Federal Ministry of Health and NTD researchers from Osun State University, conducted a study to investigate the barriers to and facilitators of implementing large-scale praziquantel programs for SAC in Nigeria.[244] Funding, political will, effective leadership, beneficiaries' awareness and acceptance of the intervention, and practicalities linked to transportation and feedback are some of the main thematic areas of barriers and facilitators identified in the study.[244] According to the data from the

WHO, Tanzania is the second-most schistosomiasis-infected African country, with an estimated 16 million people requiring treatment as of 2020.[234] Both urogenital and intestinal schistosomiasis are endemic in the country, with intestinal schistosomiasis particularly prevalent around the lake zone, where prevalence rates of up to 100% have been documented.[245] Tanzania's government has undertaken efforts to combat schistosomiasis in the country. As early as 1986, a control program for schistosomiasis was initiated on the island of Pemba.[246] The initiative's plan of action includes training health assistants to conduct selective population chemotherapy surveys in schools.[246]

In 2003, a new schistosomiasis control program (called Kick out Kichocho) was initiated in Unguja (also known as Zanzibar Island).[245] The program offered praziquantel treatment to school children. In 2004, the National Schistosomiasis and Soil-transmitted Helminths Control Programme (NSSCP) under the Ministry of Health and Social Welfare was established with support from the Schistosomiasis Control Initiative on the mainland part of Tanzania.[247] The school-based mass deworming treatment has covered 21 regions, according to a 2010 NSSCP report, with each region receiving one to three rounds of treatment. Millions of Tanzanian schoolchildren have received at least one to three rounds of praziquantel treatment, thanks to funding from the Bill and Melinda Gates Foundation and the Schistosomiasis Initiatives Control, as well as commitment from the Tanzanian government through the Ministry of Health and Social Welfare.[247]

The central government of Tanzania's request to local district authorities to allocate funds for schistosomiasis control, particularly for purchasing and distributing medications (praziquantel) to at-risk populations (primarily school children), was an innovative initiative.[239] In Uganda, MDA of praziquantel began in 2003 and 400,000 treatments of praziquantel were distributed that year. With the support of the Schistosomiasis Control Initiative, this treatment has been expanded to 1.5 million children annually.[237]

Praziquantel MDA Implementation Lessons for Africa

The Consolidated Framework for Implementation Research (CFIR) is a conceptual framework developed to guide the systematic assessment of implementation contexts and factors that influence effective intervention implementation.[248] In addition, the CFIR framework is known in systematic research to support implementing healthcare delivery interventions to produce actionable evaluations to improve implementation.[249] The CFIR includes five major domains (intervention characteristics, outer setting, inner setting, characteristics of individuals, and process) with 48 underlying constructs and sub-constructs associated with effective implementation.[250]

Domain 1: Intervention Characteristics

Intervention characteristics describe the inherent attributes of the intervention. Concerning the praziquantel MDA, the intervention characteristics revolved around the short shelf life, the bitter taste of the drug, and its size.

In interviews with implementers of preventative chemotherapy in Nigeria, the short shelf life of praziquantel tablets was one of the most significant issues, as the drug can be stored for only two years. It is not uncommon for tablets to expire before reaching the target population. In addition, many schools cannot use all the requested tablets, and inadequate coordination prevents tablets from being transported to other regions.

In a cross-sectional study conducted in Zanzibar, researchers assessed the praziquantel coverage in schools and communities for schistosomiasis and discovered that a section of the population in Unguja had not taken the full dosage of tablets because of difficulty swallowing large pills and fear of adverse side effects.[251]

In addition, many children are unwilling to take praziquantel because of the bitter taste of the drug; the large size of praziquantel tablets has also been cited as a barrier during school MDA in Nigeria. The lack of a precise manufacturing date sometimes is another serious issue that could lead to the distribution of expired and ineffective medication.

Domain 2: Outer Setting

The outer setting describes the external and environmental factors that influence the success of certain interventions. Two key elements of the outer setting include the impact of lack of adequate food before taking praziquantel tablets, political will, and strategic collaborations.

Concerns related to side effects (such as dizziness or vomiting) were among the most frequently cited barriers to implementation in Nigeria's school-based administration of praziquantel. Although eating food mitigates the majority of adverse side effects, food is not always available for children before administration because of socio-economic barriers. Supplying schools with food and scaling up food programs were key suggestions to avoid the adverse effects of the drug.

There are situations in which such factors have been overcome. For example, in Tanzania, to facilitate the administration process, all schools were instructed to provide porridge to the children on school-based treatment day to limit the number of potential drug-related side effects.[251] The community-wide treatment was carried out on the islands of Pemba and Unguja on 29 and 30 November 2013 by trained community drug distributors under the supervision of members of the NTD Control Program of the Zanzibar Ministry of Health and district health management teams.[251] The community drug distributors gave praziquantel to everyone in the Pemba and Unguja islands through a door-to-door approach. The treatment coverage data revealed school-based treatment coverage rates of 63.9% in Unguja and 84.4% in Pemba, and community-wide treatment coverage rates of 80.6% in Unguja and 82.0% in Pemba.[251] The WHO, in partnership with Merck, donated praziquantel tablets for MDAs while the Schistosomiasis Control Initiative provided funds.

A crucial lesson learned from the MDA program's successful implementation was using a customized implementation and delivery strategy to achieve the target treatment coverage. During the MDA program, both fixed posts (school-based treatment) and door-to-door treatment procedures (community-wide treatment) were used. The plan for schools to provide food for students was a great initiative that increased students' praziquantel intake.

Regarding government ownership and strategic collaborations, since 2012 in Malawi, the National Schistosomiasis Control Program has held annual MDA campaigns in every district of Malawi to administer praziquantel. In 2018, the MDA program implemented in the country targeted SAC in all districts. Preventive chemotherapy (praziquantel) was administered to SAC children in schools, children who did not attend school, and people in high-risk communities. A multi-sectoral team led by NTD and school health and nutrition coordinators from the Ministries of Health and Education implemented the MDA program. Health surveillance assistants distributed the drug in the community with the support of teachers in schools and community volunteers in villages.[252]

Health workers from the district and health centres were in charge of monitoring and supervising MDA distribution. Approximately 9.1 million people required preventive chemotherapy for schistosomiasis, and about 7.2 million were treated. A 79.2% national treatment coverage rate was achieved in Malawi, compared with the national treatment coverage rate of 44.5% in 2017.[234]

Although the MDA program was primarily the responsibility of the Ministry of Health through the National Schistosomiasis Control

Program, several partners worked with the Ministry of Health and supported the program. The cooperation for the MDA program at the national level included the Ministry of Education, Schistosomiasis Control Initiative, and Development Media International. At the district level, partners such as the German Agency for International Cooperation in Chiradzulu, Save the Children in Zomba, and the Blantyre Institute of Community Outreach in Mangochi supported the districts by providing various resources such as transportation and meals for students during the implementation of MDA.[252]

Partnering for praziquantel MDA with external organizations, ministries, and programs is an important program facilitator. In Nigeria, NGOs such as UNICEF and the Carter Foundation were crucial in providing funding, particularly remuneration for distributors. A study was conducted to identify the barriers and facilitators of the praziquantel MDA program in Nigeria.[244] Researchers interviewed key experts engaged in the MDA program to gain insights into the program's effectiveness and challenges. As mentioned by one expert, "States do not have the funds to commit to the exercise, so NGOs have been able to commit funding, funding from donors, to ensure that these medicines reach the needed population."[244] Collaborating with the Ministry of Education is particularly important for program logistics, as they can provide information regarding school enrolment, the number of primary schools within the region, and the number of classes.

Domain 3: Inner Setting

The inner setting refers to the characteristics within organizations or networks responsible for implementing the intervention. In the case of praziquantel MDA, these mainly include resources provided through school, staff support, training, and baseline data.

Administering praziquantel within schools is commonly said to be "extremely efficient," as they are centralized locations and it is "easy to get children and get people [into] one place without using a lot of resources."[244] However, frequent staff turnover can be a hindrance, as retraining teachers can be costly and time-consuming. In addition, the lack of incentives or remuneration for volunteers and teachers decreases the motivation for distribution and, thus, participation in the MDA.

Teachers are often reluctant to take on additional tasks that are beyond their full-time work responsibilities without appropriate incentives, particularly considering that MDA duties require additional training. An interviewee suggested that simply providing teachers with gifts – such as certificates, branded T-shirts, and hats – could increase participation. The acceptance and support of the MDA by school owners and staff are essential for program logistics, as schools can inform program directors of the best times for administration. For example, collaborating with school administration ensures that inconvenient times such as exam seasons or school holidays are avoided.

In Ethiopia, the first national MDA program was aimed at children ages 5 to 14. The MDA covered 61 districts across the country's 11 regions.[253] Before the campaign, health officers in each district were instructed on how to carry out the administration process and how to train healthcare workers and teachers.[254] Two weeks before the administration of praziquantel to SAC, the woreda (district) health officers trained two teachers from each school and one health professional from each kebele (smaller administrative unit of a district) for three days.[254] Lists of enrolled SAC to be treated were obtained from the school register, while non-enrolled SAC were treated by community mobilization at the nearest administering centre.

The Ethiopian government's ownership of the MDA program was a major factor. The generous donation of praziquantel tablets by the WHO contributed to the program's success. Additionally, financial, technical, and logistical support from various partners, such as the Imperial College London Schistosomiasis Control Initiative and the Children's Investment Fund Foundation, played a major role in the program's success. Finally, the intensified supervision of the drug distribution by the WHO Ethiopia Country Office and the program's flexibility in treating both enrolled and non-enrolled SAC are critical lessons learned from the MDA implementation program.[253]

The WHO Ethiopia Country Office provided technical support in training drug distributors and supervision of the drug distributors in all regions.[253] Over 5 million SAC were treated against schistosomiasis by the end of the MDA campaign, resulting in a treatment coverage of 77.7%.[255]

Concerning adequate resources, factors such as quantity of drugs, storage, human resources, training, and data management tools can be both barriers to and facilitators of the implementation process. Sometimes, the supply of praziquantel is inadequate to cover all hotspots within an MDA campaign, and without adequate storage systems and distribution channels, much of the stock will likely expire before it is used.

In addition, adequate prevalence or baseline data is necessary before schools can receive sufficient quantities of praziquantel. Thus, a statistics gap could prevent accurate drug requests from being made. Prevalence data are presented to the WHO to justify the amounts of praziquantel requested and are shared with policymakers at all levels to seek funding from international donors.

Domain 4: Characteristics of Individuals

This characteristics of individuals domain describes the factors related to individual beneficiaries that interfere with the success of certain interventions. In this case, it was mostly due to individual beliefs about praziquantel.

Lack of individual compliance is also a major barrier. Parents often express resistance to the administration of praziquantel because of distrust of Western medicine. A monitoring and evaluation officer involved in praziquantel MDA in Nigeria explained that some parents were hesitant to allow their children to take the drug, fearing it was part of a Western plot to "eliminate or sterilize them."[244]

In Tanzania, rumours of child fatalities and fainting episodes and illnesses in children following treatment fuelled speculation that the drugs were faulty, counterfeit, previously untested on humans, or part of a covert sterilization campaign.[256] A rumour about children dying after taking the drug sparked a riot in the primary schools where the MDA program was being implemented in 2008. After hearing rumours, parents and guardians rushed to primary schools to locate their children and prevent them from taking the drug.[256] Teachers were physically assaulted as parents argued and fought with them. Even the children who had previously used the drugs were visibly distressed and worried that they would die. The Ministry of Health had to officially suspend the MDA program that same day.[256]

In Kenya, a national school health policy and a national multi-year strategic plan for the control of NTDs were created in 2011, calling for preventive chemotherapy treatment to be given to all SAC based on the prevalence and severity of schistosome infection in Kenya, with the goal of decreasing infection rates to less than 1%.[257]

At the national level, the program trained master trainers who are personnel from Ministries of Health and Education based in the implementing counties. Master trainers from the county trained sub-county and division-level workers on how to manage and implement the MDA program, and they also trained teachers on how to implement a successful Deworming Day. Community sensitization and mobilization began immediately after teacher training; community-level health workers and teachers shared key messages with community members, such as children, parents, and village elders, before treatment.[258] The goal was to encourage community members to bring their children for deworming, particularly non-enrolled children. The Evidence Action Development Initiative monitoring, learning, and information systems team monitored praziquantel tablet administration in schools, and national health and education professionals also made observation visits to the schools.[259] In 2017, the National School-Based Deworming Programme treated 519,232 SAC for schistosomiasis against a target of 768,466, a 68% treatment coverage.[259]

Through various community mobilization channels, such as interpersonal communication and mass media and information, education, and communication materials targeted at parents, teachers, and children, children who were not enrolled in school were encouraged to participate in the MDA program. The impact of the program was monitored by the Kenya Medical Research Institute. The National School-Based Deworming Programme was one of Kenya's first programs to be successfully executed in the setting of devolved government institutions, as stated in the 2010 constitution and implemented in 2013. Officials from the Ministry of Health and the Ministry of Education coordinated the effort at the national level.

Domain 5: Process

The process domain describes the essential and logistical activities of implementation. Elements of this domain include difficulty accessing hard-to-reach regions and engagement with key parties.

Delivering supplies to rural or riverine areas is challenging, given the poor road conditions. However, transportation such as trucks, bikes, or even boats provided by NGOs or state governments can be beneficial to expedite MDA efforts. Passionate and committed personnel can also assist with distribution in hard-to-reach areas. Thus, adequate coordination and planning are the first steps to ensuring a smooth implementation.

Furthermore, at times, difficulty engaging partners, distributors, and unregistered students poses challenges during the implementation process. One key party involved in praziquantel MDA in Nigeria cited complex training logistics as a barrier, whereby it is difficult to "train all the layers" of teachers, distributors, and program administrators at federal, state, local, and school levels.[244] However, engaging personnel such as local kingpins or tribal leaders during implementation can directly influence individual acceptance and uptake. Three other participants cited that involving specialized personnel such as diplomatic access agents, shipping clearance workers, and security agents assisted in praziquantel MDA and that having a good relationship with shipping clearance agents is key in ensuring that the requisite drugs can enter the country smoothly.

A lack of community awareness and knowledge is another commonly cited barrier that decreases individual acceptance of the drug and can often spread misinformation. One interviewee described how some individuals do not believe in pharmaceuticals and throw away pills because they prefer traditional healing methods. Therefore, advocacy or promotional materials are essential for creating awareness regarding the benefits of praziquantel.

In Ghana, with the completion of schistosomiasis mapping in 2010, approximately 6.6 million SAC in all 170 districts were identified as being at risk.[260] The Neglected Tropical Diseases Program (NTDP) in Ghana began treating SAC with preventive chemotherapy (praziquantel) in 2008.[260]

The country held its MDA program for 2014 in November. A month before the program, the NTDP organized a national workshop to train the master trainers. With the support of the FHI 360 staff (individuals who work with government agencies and NGOs to improve Ghana's education system and support public and private health systems and services in the country), the regional and district-level training was conducted.

Community outreach was carried out in Ghana to reach out to all SAC.[261] Community outreach was needed to invite the families of children who do not attend school to come to the local school for their children's treatment. Also, the NTDP used multiple communication channels to ensure that the messages reached everyone and were clearly understood.[261]

The NTDP used different communication methods to ensure that everyone in the country was aware of the program. Parents and teachers association gatherings, church and mosque groups, and neighbourhood radio stations publicized the MDA program. In addition, the program information was broadcast to the community via mobile vans equipped with public address systems.[261]

In Ghana, during the MDA program in 2014, monitoring teams were established at the national, regional, and district levels as part of the NTDP. During the administration period, monitoring teams visited schools and communities. The regional and district-level teams handled the few reported cases of drug side effects such as dizziness, weakness, and stomach ache.[261]

Conclusion

The implementation of praziquantel highlights that an abundance of options for improvement may be available, through both course correction of ongoing program delivery and rebalancing of priorities in planned programs or extensions and later phases. The key factors in praziquantel MDA organized according to the CFIR domains can be used to build knowledge on how to adapt praziquantel MDA to national and local settings. The domains for the CFIR contain important critical factors that both prevent and assist the distribution of praziquantel in Africa and can inform successful program development and implementation.

5
Biotech Crops: To Trust or Not to Trust

Science and technology coupled with improved human capital have been powerful drivers of positive change in the performance and evolution of smallholder systems.

– Food & Agriculture Organization of the United Nations

Biotech crops have had a complex implementation process in Africa. Between 2010 and 2012, I had face-to-face interviews with more than 200 key participants across Burkina Faso, Kenya, Nigeria, Mozambique, South Africa, Tanzania, and Uganda. These people came from a variety of institutions and groups related to the agricultural biotechnology sector in the region (such as research institutes, universities, food companies, processors, farmers' associations, media houses, national agricultural research institutes, agricultural extension services, agricultural commercialization enterprises, NGOs, regulatory authorities, and seed companies).

The key objective of the interviews was to understand the factors associated with implementing biotech crops in Africa. Fourteen factors emerged from the interviews: limited public understanding; elitist media reporting; ineffective information sharing by scientists; inaccurate portrayal by NGOs, lobbyists, and civil organizations against genetically modified (GM) crops; tangible benefits and quality products; product regulation and control of traditional and GM varieties; gender roles; changing traditional practices related to farming; cultural norms related to food; playing God; local product development; distrust of the private sector; training and expertise; and legal framework. We grouped these factors into four main themes: communication, commercialization, culture and religion, and capacity building.[262]

The results demonstrated the complex nature of implementation and the significance that the issue of trust plays in biotech crop development in Africa.

This chapter briefly explores the history of biotech crops in Africa, discusses its impact, and the lessons gleaned from how trust functions in its implementation in the region.

Biotech Crops in Africa

In 1998, South Africa became the first African country to produce biotech crops commercially.[263] Scientists championed this achievement as they first brought the government's attention to novel genetic biotechnologies and then guided the government and industry by establishing a voluntary advisory committee in 1978.[263] Then, in early 1990, when the first Bt cotton (genetically modified pest-resistant cotton) trials were to be conducted, the South African Genetic Experimentation committee produced a biosafety booklet.[263] The approved document, along with the *Agricultural Plant Pests Act* and other regulations, helped with safely handling genetically modified organisms (GMOs).[263] Ultimately, the *GMO Act* was drafted by the Department of Agriculture and approved by Parliament in 2007, after GMO regulatory developments were monitored around the world.[263] Being involved in biotechnology research and development, South Africa generated a globally competitive biotechnology industry, with first-generation biotechnologies and competitive animal- and plant-breeding capabilities.[264]

Within the next decade, biotech crops were being produced in several developing countries, and in 2008, Burkina Faso and Egypt became the first West and North African countries, respectively, to commercially grow biotech crops, with Sudan following in 2012 and Eswatini doing so in 2018.[265] When Sudan and Eswatini first planted biotech crops, both countries started with Bt cotton.[265] The year after Eswatini planted Bt cotton, the number of African countries growing biotech crops doubled, and at the end of the year, 11 African countries sought regulatory approval for biotech crops.[266] The same year, in 2019, South Africa was the largest producer of biotech crops globally.[264] The year 2019 was characterized by increased awareness, acceptance, and adoption of biotech crops in Africa, which has aided advancements in biotech crop research, regulation, and adoption, and progression from field trials to environmental release.[265] This occurred because in 2019, African farmers developed greater awareness of and appreciation for biotech crops.[265] This resulted in a doubling of the number of African countries that were planting biotech crops from three in 2018 to six in 2019.[265]

Together, South Africa, Sudan, Malawi, Nigeria, Eswatini, and Ethiopia planted 2.9 million hectares of biotech crops, contributing to the global biotech crop area of 190.4 million hectares.[265] And 2019 was also the year of several achievements as Nigeria approved Bt cowpea, Kenya approved biotech crop commercialization, and Mozambique and Kenya shifted from confined field trials to environmental release of biotech crops.[265] In addition, Ghana and Niger enhanced their biosafety regulations for biotech crop development and adoption, and Zambia supported the food safety of biotech crops while promoting their trade.[265]

Impact of Biotech Crops in Africa

The most scaled-up biotech crops in Africa are Bt cotton, Bt maize, and Bt soybean.[267] South Africa was the first African country to commercialize biotech crops in 1998, starting with insect-resistant cotton. For 10 years, it was the only African country to grow biotech crops.[263] In 2016, South Africa planted 9000 hectares of biotech cotton, and in 2017, this number reached 37,406 hectares.[267] The country also experienced a growth of 315% in biotech cotton area in 2017, with 100% adoption of biotech cotton.[267] Key players are the Department of Agriculture and its GMO Secretariat, and the Executive Council, composed of Agriculture, Environment, Labour, Health, Trade and Industry, and Science and Technology.[267] A scientific team of 10 experts, as well as the GMO Advisory Committee (AC) and its subcommittee, are also crucial for the biosafety assessments of application documentation.[267] To reach consensus regarding the approval of applications, the AC presents its opinion to the Official Executive Committee, the chairman, and senior representatives of six government departments.[267]

After South Africa, Burkina Faso was the 2nd country on the African continent, and 10th country globally, to grow biotech cotton in 2008.[263] Burkina Faso's cotton industry is well organized because of collaboration between partners, like the government and cotton companies.[264] In the first year of commercialization, Burkina Faso planted around 475,000 hectares of Bt cotton.[264] However, its production was suspended in 2016 as companies raised concerns regarding the shorter length of crop fibres, which led to lower market prices.[268] As a result, researchers have been working to introduce the Bt gene into local cotton with long fibres.[269]

Another biotech crop was Bt maize in South Africa. In 2018, out of the 2.3 million hectares of maize in South Africa, 1.53 million, or 66%, was insect-resistant biotech maize.[270] Egypt was the second African country, and the first in the Arab world, to plant 700 hectares of Bt maize in

2008.[264] However, Bt maize production was halted in Egypt because of a lack of biosafety laws governing the production and commercialization of biotech crops.[268]

When Burkina Faso and Egypt commercialized biotech crops for the first time in 2008, they were two of the three countries that had commercialized biotech crops that year.[264] Having a leading country commercialize biotech crops in the three principal regions of Africa was a great accomplishment, because in 2009, Africa was struggling with its biggest challenge thus far regarding the adoption and acceptance of biotech crops.[264]

In Africa, numerous resource-poor and small-scale farmers adopted biotech crops for their effective pest control characteristics, higher yield, improved nutrition, fewer labour requirements, and reduced chemical costs, among other characteristics.[264] Since the crops are pest resistant, spraying decreased from 10 to 4 events per season in Africa, resulting in 42% less spending and a reduction in greenhouse gas emissions.[264,271]

Decreased pesticide spraying has also been associated with increased income and yield for farmers, higher global production and trading, and balanced world crop prices, with farmers in developing countries benefiting the most.[272] For example, South Africa's farm income increased by USD 156 million between 1998 and 2006, and it was estimated that an approximately 30% increase in yield could produce benefits of over USD 100 million per year.[273] Furthermore, since 2008, commercial biotech cotton production has generated jobs for 2 million to 4 million farmers in Burkina Faso.[274]

On a global level, biotech crops accounted for USD 7 billion in economic benefits in 2006 and USD 33.8 billion in an 11-year period.[272] In addition, by using biotech crops, farmers required less land for cultivation, and savings in time and money allowed women and children to dedicate themselves to their family and education.[264,275]

How Trust Functions in Biotech Implementation

In the developing world, there has been mistrust between public and private sectors and controversy around the use of GM crops, hindering the development and effectiveness of biotech public-private partnerships.[276,277] For example, Europe's strong stance against biotech crops, formed from a mistrust of government regulatory agencies and the involvement of corporations as the first biotech crop developers, among other factors, has influenced Africa's attitude as well.[278] This occurred because of Europe's aid, trade, and education involvement with Africa.[278] The European Parliament's decision to remove from the market in 2020 all biotech crops that offered antibiotic resistance negatively impacted the import of biotech crops.[278]

As a result of this decision, farmers in Africa have been hesitant to produce biotech maize for fear they cannot export it to Europe.[278] Some African countries, particularly Zambia, Mozambique, Malawi, Zimbabwe, Swaziland, and Lesotho, rejected food aid in 2002, despite having a starving population, because the food was genetically modified.[278] The food was donated by the United States, and there was suspicion that the United States was using the food crisis to promote biotechnology in Southern Africa and create dependency on US-based multinational companies.[278] The six nations believed that such a dependency would weaken local production capacity and worsen food insecurity.[278] Thus, trust is necessary for the efficiency, sustainability, and success of partnerships in agricultural biotechnology, particularly in initiatives led by public-private partnerships.[279]

A series of studies captured important conclusions from more than 80 interviews with key people in eight African agbiotech (agricultural biotechnology) projects spanning seven countries: Burkina Faso, Egypt, Kenya, Nigeria, South Africa, Tanzania, and Uganda. The insights from this five-year study into what built or undermined trust in eight African case studies were published as a supplement consisting of eight peer-reviewed articles in the UK-based journal *Agriculture and Food Security*, titled *Fostering Innovation through Building Trust: Lessons from Agricultural Biotechnology Partnerships in Africa*.[280] For example, trust can affect motivation, involvement in a partnership, and action and progression towards project goals and phases,[279] and public trust is crucial for the adoption of biotech crops.[281] Efforts to pursue trust have encouraged the implementation of good agronomic practices, ensuring the sustained effectiveness of GM technologies and improving the public's ability to trust the technology and its providers.[279,282,283]

In Africa, farm walks conducted with Bt cotton in Burkina Faso and Bt maize in Egypt allowed participants to observe the field activities of public-private partnerships and compare the performance of biotech crops and conventional crops.[283] Such engagement is an effective method of fostering trust.[279] Trust leads to better performance and productivity[282] and saves time and money.[284] All these factors combined have ultimately facilitated the development and scale of biotech crops in Africa. Six critical determinants of trust in implementing agbiotech programs are honesty (and integrity), accountability, capability (and competency), solidarity or the same vision, transparency, and generosity (humanitarianism).[285]

Element 1: Honesty and Integrity

Honesty is an essential criterion for establishing trust. All partners involved in agbiotech projects must be truthful about what they can promise and deliver, especially to the public, and what the agricultural technology can and cannot do, as well as the health risks posed by the technology. All partners must be truthful in all communications. It is also important not to over-promise; promises that will be difficult to fulfil should be avoided.

Regarding Bt maize in South Africa, on-farm demonstration was initiated to build trust between farmers and the private sector. Monsanto (then an American agrochemical and agricultural biotechnology corporation) launched the on-farm demonstration practice in South Africa in 2001 to engage farmers by holding workshops across the country.[283] The initiative aimed to introduce Bt maize to over 3000 small-scale farmers. During the on-farm demonstration, seed companies or distributors gave farmers free Bt and conventional maize seeds to plant in sections of their fields to compare crop performance and yield. Farmers were also compensated for hosting field days and inviting other farmers in the community to observe the differences in performance at the demonstration sites. Individuals who participated in demonstrations described them as trust-building practices because of the support that seed companies and AfricaBio provided to farmers regarding seed supply, labour compensation, and technology education. The primary goal of these on-farm demonstrations was to build trust among participating farmers, who could compare the performance of Bt maize to traditional maize first-hand.[283]

However, individuals who had hosted on-farm demonstrations described the erosion of trust that occurred when seed companies or distributors withheld or failed to fulfil promises of financial compensation for their efforts. Because of the lack of compensation, some farmers have stated that they will no longer host field days and crop demonstrations.[283] According to the farmers, they used to trust AfricaBio and the private seed companies because of the things they were doing, but as money and input support dwindled, trust dwindled as well.

In South Africa, the Department of Agriculture approved Monsanto's MON810 (a genetically modified maize) for commercial production in 1998, based on the South African Genetic Experimentation committee's recommendation. In 2003, Syngenta's Bt maize was also approved.[286] To foster trust during the regulatory approval process, both the applicant (Monsanto) and the regulator (Department of Agriculture) truthfully disclosed all relevant information.[283] The government clarified regulatory approval requirements and communicated them to private companies. According to a former regulator, who is now a seed company executive, the early stages of developing Bt maize were a learning experience for regulators that was aided by honest communication with the industry.[283]

Honest communication, truthful information, and not withholding information that could influence decision-making between the regulatory body and private companies were big factors that contributed to building trust, which in turn led to better regulatory compliance.[283] Mutual trust between the regulator and industry has resulted in improved communication and consultation. When lobbyists or anti-GMO organizations complain about Bt maize technology, the government trusts the private sector enough to approach them by saying, "This is an accusation that came in about your products. What information can you give us?" The mutual trust between regulatory bodies and the private sector facilitated this positive relationship. The guarantee that the Bt maize technology works and honesty about its expected performance were important trust-building practices.

Element 2: Results Delivery and Accountability

Building trust requires the delivery of a good and effective product or technology. In the case of South Africa's Bt maize project, trust was possible because the technology worked. The ability of the technology to increase crop yields or reduce input costs was critical to building trust in the technology.[283] A small-scale farmer who was interviewed ascertained that farmers are building trust in the Bt cotton seed itself. The performance of the seed is what they trusted, though there were times when the performance of the Bt maize technology in South Africa did not meet farmers' expectations.[283] A few of these incidents provided an opportunity to build trust, as the private companies involved accepted responsibility for product failures and compensated affected farmers. In other words, the private companies were accountable for the product failure. There were also cases in which product failures eroded trust between the farmer and the private seed company involved, with the latter refusing to acknowledge or accept responsibility for the reported discrepancies.

Failure to consistently meet deadlines, mismanagement of funds, and lack of follow-through on commitments were significant barriers to trust building in the Bt cowpea project in Nigeria.[287]

The quality of the technology product, as measured by its capacity to improve yields, is a critical foundation for establishing trust. Farmers in Egypt adopted Bt maize because the product was effective and yielded results. According to Egyptian farmers, their trust in the new product has little to do with the values and motivations of the seed companies involved and everything to do with the seed technology's ability to deliver the promised benefits to farmers.[288] In other words, positive product outcomes help to build trust between the community, specifically farmers and the technology. This supports the notion that positive first-hand experience with the seeds lays the groundwork for project partners and farmers to build trust in the technology and with one another.[288] As a result, the ability of the seed to deliver in terms of technological capacity is as significant as the motives and ideologies of corporations or organizations involved in the development of Bt maize.[288]

In Burkina Faso, a problem with the physical quality of the seeds posed a significant challenge to the project's success.[282] A technical issue of smaller seeds and poor germination emerged, affecting trust between partners and farmers. Because of this, some farmers refused to plant Bt cotton seed.[282] Farmers who rejected the Bt cotton seed emphasized that their lack of trust stemmed from the sources themselves, not the GM crop.[282] To maintain trust, seed quality must meet or exceed farmer expectations.

According to a Bt maize farmer from South Africa, trust is "when they said that they will deliver on a certain day, and they do deliver." In Kenya, the commercialization of the Insect Resistant Maize for Africa (IRMA) products was expected to begin at the end of phase II of the project, with both transgenic and conventional products becoming available to the public.[289] The end users already had high expectations for IRMA products, particularly Bt-based maize varieties. However, the community was disheartened by the failure to deliver these varieties, which raised doubts about IRMA's ability to deliver. As a result, the community's trust in the project, particularly by farmers and seed companies, was eroded.[289]

Element 3: Capability and Competency

The progress of the Bt cotton project in Burkina Faso was limited by a lack of trust and confidence in Burkinabè researchers. The widely held belief that a low-income country like Burkina Faso cannot produce high-tech goods exacerbated public scepticism about the Bt cotton project's future viability. The widespread perception of Burkinabè researchers as "incapable" and "incompetent" pervaded their interactions with international research peers.[282]

To control cotton bollworm, three East African countries (Kenya, Uganda, and Tanzania) considered using genetically modified cotton.[290] The Kenya Agricultural Research Institute (KARI) and the multinational seed company Monsanto collaborated on the project in Kenya.[290] Kenya was able to commercialize GM crops because its biosafety laws gave the country the capacity to do so. Knowing that a country can commercialize or adopt the use of genetically modified crops is critical in building trust. The positive relationship between KARI and Monsanto shed light on two factors that have contributed to their mutual trust. The first factor is that Kenya has a favourable biosafety legal framework, which allowed Monsanto to reach an agreement with KARI. Second, the technical staff was competent and dedicated. Monsanto representatives acknowledged that Uganda's National Biotechnology and Biosafety Policy provided a suitable environment for private sector engagement, serving as a foundation for trust-building practices. During the project's period in Tanzania, there was a delay caused by what the private partner perceived to be unfavourable legislation in the country, which prevented Monsanto from providing the Bt cotton technology for trials.[290] There is a need for a legal framework that encourages private sector participation and serves as a foundation for building trust. Individual country regulatory frameworks are thus required.

Element 4: Same Vision and Mutual Interest

The disparities between France and the United States in providing guidance on GM crops in Burkina Faso posed a significant challenge to building trust in the country's agbiotech projects.[282] France and the United States had opposing views on introducing genetically modified crops in Burkina Faso. As a result, the Burkinabè government was caught in the middle.[282]

The guidance provided by such external influences left the Burkinabè government unsure about how to proceed with GM crops in the country, making it more hesitant to trust the scientists at its research institutes. According to a researcher from the Institut de l'Environnement et de Recherche Agricoles (INERA), these disparities created some confusion within the government and the research institutes, which were caught between these conflicting opinions.

Element 5: Transparency

Clearly articulating motives and risks is vital in building trust in public-private partnerships. One of the main factors related to the success of the Bt cotton project in Burkina Faso was the open disclosure of institutional motivations early in the projects. Several partner meetings were held to ensure that partners felt comfortable disclosing their motivations, including profit-making motives. This practice increased transparency by allowing partners to communicate, reducing suspicions and increasing trust.[282]

One issue emerged as a barrier to trust building: the public discourse surrounding GM products was based on incorrect information. The false information included the belief that GM foods cause allergies and sterility. Furthermore, activists and intellectuals were strongly opposed to the project because of a lack of reliable, scientifically supported information on Bt cotton.[282]

The lack of transparency and accurate information reaching civil society groups and the public resulted in lower levels of trust. To dispel misconceptions about GM products, the Bt cotton project launched a communication campaign, which included the Seeing is Believing seminars. Members of the public were invited to the test fields during these workshops.[282] The Seeing is Believing seminars allowed the public to visit the Bt cotton trial sites and witness the cotton's growth. The initiative was effective in building trust in the project.[282]

In the case of the Bt cotton projects in East Africa, during the project, all financial issues were openly discussed among project partners to ensure transparency and trust.[290] Information generated by partners was shared and communicated among project partners via phone calls and exchange visits, all of which contributed to the development of trust.[290] A free flow of information prevented research overlaps and gave scientists independence and confidence in one another. A Makerere University academic described the practice of sharing information and resources as an accountable and collaborative approach that increased trust.[290]

Element 6: Humanitarianism

The goal of agricultural biotechnology is to benefit the public rather than to make a profit. Monsanto attempted to engage farmers in 2001 by holding nine workshops across South Africa to introduce over 3000 small-scale farmers to Bt maize.[283] Each farmer received two bags of seed, one of Bt maize and one of conventional maize, to plant in their fields to compare crop performance and yield.[286] As noted, farmers were also compensated for hosting field days and inviting other farmers in the community to observe the differences in performance at the demonstration sites.[283]

This practice was used in six demonstration plots organized by AfricaBio between 2004 and 2005, and the results showed that Bt maize yields were higher because of reduced stem borer infestations compared with conventional maize.[291] The primary goal of these on-farm demonstrations was to build trust among participating farmers, who were able to compare the performance of Bt maize and traditional maize first-hand.[283]

Summary

Trust is arguably the most crucial issue regarding the challenges and complexities surrounding Africa's arduous scale-up of biotech crops. Critical lessons for scaling up biotech crops are delineated through the lens of trust, drawing from varied examples in Burkina Faso, Egypt, Kenya, Nigeria, South Africa, Tanzania, and Uganda. Biotech crop scale-up in Africa provides a view into the importance of trust and how it functions, which can inform practical actions and has policy implications for scaling up technologies. The theoretical and practical implications of focusing on trust in implementing biotech crops are encapsulated through six critical determinants: honesty (and integrity), accountability, capability (and competency), solidarity or the same vision, transparency, and generosity (humanitarianism).

6
Vitamin A Has a Story to Tell

Vitamin A supplements can improve a child's chance of survival by 12 to 24 percent.[292]

Vitamin A deficiency is considered one of the most prevalent micronutrient deficiencies across the globe, and in 2020, it was reported that only 41% of targeted children received vitamin A supplementation, with West and Central Africa reporting the lowest coverage (29%).[53] The COVID-19 pandemic negatively impacted vitamin A supplementation (VAS) programs in Africa; however, the decline in VAS coverage occurred even before the pandemic.[53,293,294]

What are the key implementation challenges to VAS, and how can they be overcome? Using the backdrop of the historical context of VAS in Africa, this chapter delineates key lessons in fostering more effective VAS in the region.

Vitamin A was first discovered in the early 1930s to be involved in the vision cycle of the retina; this finding was essential in understanding the relationship between vitamin A consumption and certain ocular diseases.[295]

Vitamin A is an essential nutrient for the human body and is crucial in maintaining the visual, physiological, and immunological systems.[296] The human body does not produce vitamin A, so its daily intake is required to prevent any adverse health outcomes from micronutrient deficiency.[296,297] The WHO[298] estimates that approximately 190 million children under five years of age are affected by vitamin A deficiency (VAD).

In the 1960s, the WHO conducted the first global survey of xerophthalmia, leading to the discovery that VAS was essential in preventing it.[299] In 1975, an organization called the International Vitamin A

Consultive Group (IVCAG) began to lead research in VAD disorders to create evidence-based programs involving treatments such as VAS.[300]

The vehicles for vitamin A programs can vary depending on the affected population. For example, food-based approaches such as food fortification and consumption of foods rich in vitamin A are more feasible for a population living in a large geographic area.[301] VAS is another type of vitamin A program, in which vitamin A is given to at-risk populations who are suffering from VAD.[301] Another approach is the use of high-dose supplements for children ages 6 to 59 months.[301,302] The WHO works with local governments to implement the use of these high-dose capsules for children in this age group. A study in Indonesia has examined the use of capsules for the supplementation of vitamin A in children.[303] Capsules with vitamin A were given to preschool children, and recipients of the capsules presented with decreased VAD compared with non-recipients.[303]

In the early stages of VAS research during the 1970s, the IVCAG and WHO focused their research on how vitamin A can prevent blindness and other ocular diseases. There was a shift in focus when several studies in the early 1990s demonstrated significant improvements in overall morbidity and mortality rates from VAS because of vitamin A's role in maintaining immune function.[304] As a result, VAS became more widespread through the WHO's introduction of specific guidelines and non-profit organizations, like Helen Keller Intl, creating VAS programs within local communities.[305]

UNICEF[292] emphasizes that vitamin A supplements can improve a child's survival rate by 12 to 24 percent. UNICEF actively supports national VAS programs in more than 80 priority countries as a critical child survival intervention. Strategies such as fortifying food and improving dietary diversity are crucial for ending VAD over the long term; however, until such programs are sustained at scale, VAS programs are essential to ensure child survival today.[292]

Impact of VAS

VAS was first implemented in research trials by Dr. Mclaren[306] during the early 1960s in India and Jordan. He concluded that VAS can prevent blindness that is caused by VAD disorders. The programs were officially implemented in the 1990s as there was strong research supporting VAS improving mortality and morbidity rates during childhood.[300] Keith West, Alfred Sommer, and Gregory Hussey are notable researchers who conducted control trials in the 1990s investigating the relationship between VAS and mortality rates.[307,308] These control trials were then used in meta-analyses, like one conducted in 1993 by Wafaie Fawzi, which demonstrated consistency in the effectiveness of VAS.[309]

Extensive research has been conducted from the 1980s to the present day supporting the efficacy of VAS. A systematic review of 47 studies that analyzed the effectiveness of VAS found that there were significant reductions in mortality and morbidity rates of children between 6 and 59 months of age after biannual supplementation.[310] According to several additional meta-analyses and systematic reviews on VADs, VAS has specifically been shown to reduce deaths related to measles, diarrheal diseases, and respiratory infections, which are common causes of death among children in developing countries.[311,312] Sub-Saharan Africa currently has a child mortality rate of 73 per 1000 live births, which is one of the highest rates globally. Providing countries within Africa with VAS is necessary as VAD currently accounts for a significant portion of child mortality.[313] Considering VAS can reduce death caused by diarrheal diseases, which are one of the leading causes of child mortality in Africa, this program has had a very positive impact.

Previous systematic reviews have looked at the direct health outcomes of vitamin A programs on populations at risk of VAD.[296] Additional reviews determined that VAS reduces mortality and morbidity for children under the age of five.[312] Investigations into how micronutrients, specifically vitamin A monitoring and supplementation, could be applied to a global scale have also been conducted.[314] However, these papers were unable to clearly distinguish the barriers and facilitators to vitamin A programs. The reviews also tended to focus narrowly on a specific type of intervention or country rather than an overall perspective globally. For example, a review conducted in Bangladesh summarized VAD. The review highlighted the lack of research on vitamin A fortification over three decades, with only a limited number of studies investigating dietary intakes in specific populations, including in young children.[315] By understanding dietary intake and current prevalence of VAD, strategies can be implemented to best meet the needs of specific populations. In addition, there have been drops in vitamin A programs[316] and vitamin A program implementation research.

Scaling Up VAS

Globally, many countries that once had a successful vitamin A delivery system are losing those platforms in part because of the phasing out of polio immunization.[317] Since children receiving VAS during polio immunization was a common strategy, eradication of polio has affected VAS.[317] The decrease in funding for polio immunization following eradication also impacted VAS, which relied on the co-financing of polio immunization.[317]

In 2016 alone, the global coverage of a two-dose vitamin A program dropped to 64%, the lowest it had been in 6 years,[317] and data from 2017 suggested that this coverage trend continued.[318] There are many reasons why, but weak health systems and sustainability are the most significant problems. Communities suffering from weak health systems and infrastructure, such as distance from health facilities like those in Africa and South Asia, are unable to reach the most vulnerable groups, especially children.[317] Sustainability is also an issue when countries face challenges in maintaining long-term coverage rates as a result of limited funding and lack of national planning.[317]

Current trends identified in the literature point to the importance of identifying the barriers to and facilitators of the implementation of vitamin A programs. The identification of these factors aids in developing programs that consider continuing constraints and mediators, with the goal of addressing the drops in coverages and ensuring long-term sustainability. There have been calls for a renewed focus in light of the COVID-19 pandemic.[294,316]

Scaling Up VAS in Africa

The IVCAG (now called the Nutrient Forum) and the WHO were crucial players in spreading VAS globally, starting in the 1970s, especially in sub-Saharan Africa, which had some of the highest rates of VAD. With USAID's help, they researched VAD and the effectiveness of VAS through controlled trials.[307] By the 1990s, there was significant literature supporting its effectiveness with VAD disorders and its ability to reduce overall child mortality rates. From here, the WHO worked on guidelines surrounding VAS programs to help implement them globally. Numerous other organizations currently lead and fund VAS programs in Africa, including Nutrition International and Helen Keller International.[319]

With solid evidence supporting the efficacy of VAS and key health organizations such as the WHO pushing for VAS programs within developing countries, VAS quickly gained traction and spread throughout the world. After the implementation of VAS in 1992, researchers generated additional evidence while observing the efficacy of the intervention in decreasing mortality rates in children, demonstrating improvements in the health of children enrolled in this program.[320] With consistent evidence supporting this intervention, VAS prevalence and recognition snowballed globally.[321]

VAD was one of the leading micronutrient deficiencies in Africa, estimated to have affected over 30 million children in 2009.[322] VAD was also found to be much more common in children affected by malaria, although it's unclear whether VAD is aggravated by malaria or if VAD somehow increases the likelihood of infection. Regardless, if a child also has VAD, they're more likely to have malaria complications because of vitamin A's role in immune system function.[322] Because of the prevalence of VAD within sub-Saharan Africa, as well as vitamin A's connection to improving the outcome of malaria, VAS programs were introduced. Since the introduction of VAS in 1990 and numerous other health initiatives, there has been a significant decrease in child mortality rates in Africa.[323] In 2019 alone, there was an estimated reduction of between 12% and 24% in child mortality in sub-Saharan Africa, preventing the deaths of an estimated 140,000 children.[324]

All countries within sub-Saharan Africa, excluding three (Gabon, Benin, and Guinea-Bissau), have implemented VAS. In 2018, it was estimated that an average of 65% of children between 6 months and 5 years were covered. However, there has been a substantial decrease in the coverage of VAS within sub-Saharan Africa since 2010.[325] While this may seem alarming, a decrease in VAS may not cause an increase in VAD disorders as there have been vast improvements in dietary diversification and the fortification of foods with vitamin A.[300] Recent research found that VAS in Burkina Faso, Nigeria, and Kenya is not as cost-effective as it was, which is likely due to an overall decrease in VAD within these countries.[326] In Gabon's case, it is one of the three countries that had no VAS coverage in 2018, despite VAD being a significant public health issue; the effects of VAD emerged in ocular vision issues and delayed growth in Gabonese children.[327]

In 2020, because of COVID-19, it was estimated that 100 million children globally missed at least one VAS dose; a large number of these children were likely from sub-Saharan Africa.[328] Despite the yearly improvements in child mortalities in Africa, stopping VAS programs is dangerous as many children (estimated to be around 43.2 million children in 2005) are still deficient in vitamin A.[329] Currently, there is inequity in action with children who do not receive VAS treatments. Various factors are associated with the likelihood a child will receive VAS, such as the mother's age, education, residence, occupational status, and media exposure, and the age of the child. Focusing on nutritional knowledge, factors that increase maternal nutritional knowledge, such as higher education and age, could also increase the awareness of the benefits of VAS, which would increase the likelihood a mother would bring her child to a VAS program. Women in sub-Saharan Africa with higher education were more likely to bring their children to a VAS program. In addition, children with older mothers were also more likely to receive VAS.[330]

Rural areas generally have lower VAS coverage because of a lack of understanding of the subject matter and logistical challenges – for example, people in hard-to-reach places may not know the program exists. Zimbabwe, one of the countries with a VAS program, is an example of a country in which rural communities have lower VAS rates. A group of researchers decided to conduct outreach within a specific rural community and increased coverage from less than 50% to 71%.[331] These findings demonstrate the importance of ensuring VAS campaigns are visible and accessible to all populations, as inequity will only impede progress in improving global health. VAS programs remain relevant in improving children's health in African countries.

Implementation Lessons

Lesson 1: Operational Management Is Vital

The first step in operational management is the adequacy and accuracy of data on the extent of VAD, which are essential for VAS programs. Accurate and complete data allow policymakers and community leaders to understand where the population stands on VAD, whether targets are being reached, and whether programs should be scaled up or down. Countries that have made sustained efforts to combat VAD have succeeded because of the increased awareness and availability of epidemiological information.[332] However, just as increased accuracy of VAD data can improve implementation, outdated data can result in program failures. Examining global VAD, a study found that most nationally representative data on vitamin status were indeed outdated, with most VAD data more than 10 years old.[304] Outdated data does not account for changing micronutrient trends and conditions in developing countries. Therefore, current national data are required to make appropriate evidence-based decisions. VAD prevalence needs to be assessed regularly to account for changing consumption patterns, which will help by reducing costs. Accurate data can allow programs to be more precise in their targeting. This is a crucial step in identifying the prevalence of VAD by location and, thus, making the appropriate allocation of resources during the implementation process to areas with VAD.

Data must be collected at the subnational level, integrated into program design, and combined with regular quality assessment and systematic data collection during implementation to reassess and adjust. Monitoring and assessments are essential for successful implementation as they provide the vital data required to guide further program planning. They also help assign and reallocate resources more efficiently if necessary.

With knowledge of the adequacy and accuracy of data on the extent of VAD, the next step is developing plans and evaluation mechanisms, which are necessary components of a successful program. A common barrier to VAS is deficits in operational planning, which can manifest in the following problems: accurate determination of age,[333] evaluation mechanisms,[334] and capsule expiration before consumption.[335] For example, the expiration of vitamin A capsules before consumption was a challenge to the VAS program in South Africa.[335] A good stock control practice is essential to ensure sufficient vitamin A capsules and prevent capsule expiration before consumption.[335] In Mali, determining children's age and classifying them into targeted groups was important.[333] Without it, children older than 59 months could have mistakenly been included as part of the target group of children under 59 months and received the supplementation.[333] This could have contributed to the low stock of vitamin A capsules experienced in Mali.[333]

In an evaluation of a VAS program in Ethiopia, constraints of programming were identified, including that "monitoring and evaluation mechanisms, which are essential components of any programme, were minimal or totally unavailable."[334(p.4)] This lack highlighted that deficits in operation planning of supplementation programs are an impediment to their use. An evaluation of the Expanded Programme on Immunisation integrated vitamin A capsule program revealed that health institutions did not submit reports and were not supervised. Only one health institution attempted to record age, date, physiological status, and dosage.

Lesson 2: More Effective Resource Mobilization Is Needed

Cost and resources are critical for sustainability. The issue of cost concerning VAS is mainly associated with a lack of financial sustainability, over-reliance on donors, and inadequate funding for programs. This is not surprising as 82% of regulatory agencies in LMICs in Africa and Asia stated that their current programs were not completely sustainable over the next five years, because of inadequate funding[336] and the high costs of VAS.[337] The lower the financial costs, the more likely the program will be sustained. For countries that are not able to sustain their vitamin A programs alone, international funding is a critical component.[337] Lack of funding was frequently cited[334,338,339] where limited budgets[334,338] and financial instability[339] restricted programs.

Stand-alone VAS programs can be double the cost of programs that are integrated with other health interventions.[337] More integrated micronutrient uptake programs can mitigate costs, which requires reviewing the comparative costs of various vitamin A programs such as supplementation, fortification, nutrition education, and other health interventions and their advantages. The high financial costs of an intervention were barriers to implementation in the vitamin A programs in Zambia.[340] A study conducted in Zambia to assess the cost-effectiveness of vitamin A interventions revealed that fortification with oil is the most cost-effective, followed by Child Health Week (an intervention in which children ages 6 to 59 months receive vitamin A capsules).[340]

Support for the vitamin A programs must include members of the community participating in implementation, funding to support programs, and high levels of advocacy to promote awareness.[334] Strong governmental support is also a factor[341,342] and can influence the uptake of VAS and the progress of programs. Support from communication and media networks on radio and television and in newspapers at both the local and national levels[333,343] remains important. Lack of program communication can be a barrier to successful implementation of VAS programs.[344] Barriers to effective communication "may have included differences in language and educational achievement, which could be difficult for a health worker to address when working in an overcrowded health facility."[344(p.40)]

Lesson 3: Knowledge and Beliefs about the Intervention Should Not Be Overlooked

The knowledge available to the population, research being done in the subject area, and information shared with staff during the implementation of the VAS programs are essential. First, parents' and caregivers' knowledge and beliefs can be a barrier to implementing VAS programs. This is evident from studies showing that caregiver knowledge significantly influenced vitamin A uptake in children.[335,345,346] Knowledge has been crucial in other vitamin and mineral supplementation programs and has a strong independent association with the use of supplements during pregnancy.[347]

Vitamin A programs need to explore knowledge awareness facilitators, which include integration with external campaigns, media communication, and media networks. These knowledge facilitators increase knowledge about and improve attitudes towards nutritional programs, as illustrated in an experimental study in Kenya that successfully used community-based health education to improve knowledge about and attitudes towards iron and folic acid supplementation among pregnant women.[348] National Nutrition Weeks in Mali were instrumental in fostering VAS. These results are not unique to vitamin A programs but are relevant to other public health nutrition programs. The linkage between knowledge and effective implementation is mirrored in wide-scale health programs such as immunization programs, where the attitudes and knowledge of mothers were associated with the vaccination status of their children. For example, in rural Uganda, mothers who understood the importance of immunization were more likely to immunize their children.[349]

Some studies have associated maternal education and VAS.[293,350,351] High levels of formal schooling education were also an influencing factor, with paternal education strongly associated with children's vitamin A coverage as well.[333] Conversely, low levels of parental education, including formal schooling for both the mother and the father, were cited as factors limiting the uptake of VAS.[352,353] Low parental awareness about supplementation programs was also cited as a barrier to implementation, as children who missed vitamin A campaigns and doses did so because the caretakers were unaware of the campaign.[335,345]

Negative attitudes and values regarding micronutrient programs have also been found to influence the success of interventions. For example, in Sokoto State in Nigeria, paternal disapproval of the intervention was a significant barrier to the uptake of VAS in the state.[351] Possible reasons for the disapproval are linked to sociocultural beliefs and suspicion that it may be harmful to the children.[351] The authors argued that this is unsurprising; the Gwadabawa local government area in Sokoto State, Nigeria, is mainly patriarchal, and men are heads of households and make decisions for the households.[351] High levels of misinformation about programs were singularly cited as a barrier.

Lesson 4: High Levels of Staff Training Facilitate Implementation

High levels of staff training result in effective distribution and coverage of VAS.[333,344] A study conducted in Mali suggested that all staff in charge of administering supplements must receive training before the event to ensure success.[333] Trained personnel are reliable, motivated, and self-assured resources for effectively performing a task. National health services and NGOs working in nutrition have extensive experience in training and supervision in Mali. The strategy implemented involves training master trainers at the national level, who then train other trainers in each health district at all other levels.[333] According to a study by du Plessis et al.,[335] 93% of nurses at primary healthcare clinics had received training from the local dietitian on VAS. As a result, no issues with implementing the VAS program in healthcare facilities were recorded.[335]

Inadequately trained staff is frequently a problem in implementing VAS and fortification programs.[344,345] Similar results were discovered in a study in Tanzania, where measurement errors in tally sheets by the health workers were observed, which resulted in discrepancies in coverage rates.[345] The large disparity in coverage rate was attributed to a variety of factors, including health workers' errors in summarizing the tally sheets. The study reported that only 32% of health workers had received any training in VAS, which is concerningly low considering that the health workers are the first point of contact in communities.[345] Furthermore, the overall nutritional knowledge of health workers was poor.[345]

Health workers must have necessary knowledge and information on VAS to improve the success of the program. Health workers should receive standardized training on the VAS program to ensure accurate data recording. In Ethiopia, for example, advocacy and sensitization activities were carried out to raise awareness among health workers through training, seminars, and the development of distribution guidelines and teaching materials.[334] However, insufficient numbers of health personnel posed a significant challenge in implementing the VAS program in Ethiopia. In a study that evaluated eight health institutions (two health centres and six clinics), three of the health clinics had only one health staff member, three had two health staff members, and only two health centres had more than two health staff members.[334] Health staff members included doctors, nurses, health assistants, and sanitarians (specialists in sanitary science and public health).[334]

Lesson 5: Adaptation of Innovation to Local Contexts

The presentation, assembly, and design of an intervention are influential factors for VAS programs. Implementers need to adapt to several local challenges, such as living in rural and pastoral terrains or the longer distances and increased travel time to community centres. For example, in Ethiopia "pastoralist communities have a dispersed settlement pattern and season mobility, which may explain the low coverage of vitamin A supplementation."[354(p.4)] Sometimes longer distances and increased travel time to community centres serve as barriers to VAS uptake.[345] Shortages in staff and supplies were additionally recognized barriers. Lack of health personnel resulted in difficulty implementing the vitamin A programs.[355,356] Disruptions in the supply chain were also highlighted as causing shortages of supplements and serving as a barrier to implementation.[343]

One study found strong procurement and distribution to be a critical determinant of program success by ensuring an adequate, timely, and sustainable supply of VAS.[357] Finally, a lack of sustainability of programs and an emphasis on short-term strategies were identified as barriers to long-term interventions.[333,358,359(p.1)]

In Ghana, having easy access to consumable capsules was found to improve VAS uptake, with the size, shape, and colour of the supplement all being contributory factors to the program's overall success.[343] The size (small), shape (round), form (transparent), and colour (honey-coloured) of the proposed vitamin A capsule were generally acceptable because it was slippery and looked easy to swallow without chewing. Appropriate packaging to reduce capsule loss, and favourable formulation such as colour and size are critical in facilitating VAS uptake.

Leveraging other programs can help with VAS. In Niger, the responsiveness and flexibility of the Ministry of Public Health were essential for making the most efficient use of resources.[360] This allowed the Ministry to take advantage of opportunities to integrate VAS into other programs, such as immunization campaigns.[360] In a study by Wirth and colleagues,[304] 82 countries were examined with varying VAS programs; in 38 countries with over 70% VAS coverage, 30 had at least one other vitamin A program in place, with over half having two or more fortified food or vitamin A programs.

Finally, programs with flexible dosing mechanisms[357] to reach all children of socially disadvantaged communities served as a facilitator for VAS.

Lesson 6: Integration with External Campaigns Works

The use of immunization programs has been effective as a VAS vehicle. The WHO and UNICEF have used immunization programs to deliver VAS to those in need.[361] Countries with VAD that have carried out immunization days for polio were encouraged to provide an appropriate oral dose of vitamin A to children ages 6 to 59 months.[361] These countries were also encouraged to add VAS to other campaigns, such as measles and tetanus eradication, especially when the campaigns focused on hard-to-reach populations at risk for VAD.[361] A study conducted by Benn et al.[362] found that VAS administered with vaccines during national immunization days in Guinea-Bissau helped improve the health outcomes of children 6 months and older, linking the use of immunization campaigns to the overall effectiveness of vitamin A programs.[361]

In two studies,[354,363] the integration of vitamin A programs with campaigns such as Day of the African Child and World AIDS Day events[363] increased facilitation, and the use of outreach strategies[354] aided in effective supplementation. In an additional study, the integration of vitamin A programs with immunization programs was a facilitator for implementation.[342] These included integration with polio immunization,[357] national immunization days,[342,346,358,364,365] and existing popular immunization programs.[340]

In Tanzania, efforts to combat VAD began in 1987 with a disease-targeted approach.[363] But many young children in Tanzanian communities at risk for VAD were reported not to have received vitamin treatments. In 1997, VAS was included as part of the Essential Drugs Programme for postpartum mothers and children at 9 months, along with measles vaccination.[363] As part of the measles vaccination campaigns in late 1999 and 2000, children between the ages of 6 and 59 months received vitamin A supplements at the same time.

VAS was strategically integrated into the Day of the African Child and World AIDS Day campaigns to increase coverage. As a result, VAS coverage in children increased from 13% in 1999 to 76% in 2002.[363] Therefore, the integration of VAS into other health campaigns can have a significant impact on coverage.

Integration with community activities was evident in three studies[355,366,367] and was observed to be a facilitator. These community activities focused on nutrition education and social mobilization[366] and using community health centres[303,367] such as the *Anganwadi*,[355] which had functional and administrative linkages with the primary health centres. The involvement of female community workers as key players in the implementation of vitamin A programs was highlighted in an additional three studies.[353,356,365]

Inadequate monitoring of programs was a barrier to successful supplementation, as was the case during the mass distribution campaigns in Tanzania, where VAS was not recorded on personal health cards.[363] Finally, it was also identified that the VAS approach that operated solely on routine health services was inadequate[354] and a barrier to effective implementation.

Summary

Myriad factors are key to successfully implementing VAS programs. Commonly reported factors in the literature and from practitioners' experience include increasing knowledge, garnering support for these programs, taking into account geographic and demographic complexities in program implementation, adapting the innovation to local settings, and monitoring operational management. With the decline in VAS programs despite evidence of rising VAD in most of Africa, the planning and design of new and ongoing evaluations and the development of implementation strategies need to be tailored to six key areas: (1) more robust operational management in VAS programs, (2) more effective resource mobilization from participants, (3) education of parents and caregivers on the importance of vitamin A, (4) high levels of staff training to facilitate implementation, (5) adaptation to effectively address geographic and demographic complexities in program implementation, and (6) integration of vitamin A programs with existing health campaigns, such as immunization programs.

7
mHealth: Spreading or Stalling?

Starting now and lasting until forever, your health and healthcare will be determined, to a remarkable and somewhat disquieting degree, by how well the technology works.

– Robert Wachter

What makes the scale-up of one mHealth initiative soar while another dies before it ever takes off? This chapter explores the emergence of mHealth innovations, their implementation and scale-up in Africa, and lessons learned from various mHealth innovations being implemented across Africa.

Robert Istepanian of London's Kingston University coined mHealth and broadly defined it as the use of "emerging mobile communications and network technologies for healthcare."[368] He is a leading authority and pioneer of mobile healthcare and served in several academic and research positions in the United Kingdom and Canada.[368]

In his book *The Digital Doctor: Hope, Hype, and Harm at the Dawn of Medicine's Computer Age*, Wachter[369] reflected on the growing influence of technology in healthcare, with the quality and accessibility of healthcare services becoming increasingly reliant on technological advancements. He hinted at a future where health outcomes may be closely connected to the efficiency and reliability of health technologies. There is also a sense of unease being communicated, because although technology may have the potential to enhance healthcare, it also introduces complexities and dependencies.

Today, mHealth includes the use of mobile communication devices, such as mobile phones, personal digital assistants, patient-monitoring devices, and other wireless devices to improve point-of-service data collection, patient communication, and distribution of emergency and routine health services.[370,371] Fiordelli et al.[372] conducted a systematic review of 117 articles and found that mHealth applications addressed mHealth research conditions such as diabetes, obesity/overweight, mental health, tobacco use, and HIV.

mHealth can be considered a subcategory of eHealth, a broader term for using all electronic technologies, such as computers, in medicine and public health.[373] As of 2012, about 75% of the world's population had access to a mobile phone, and people started using mobile phones in the early 1990s.[372] Years after the adoption of mobile phones worldwide, countries like Ethiopia, Kenya, Nigeria, and South Africa have generated several mHealth solutions, allowing them to become leaders in mobile health services usage.[375]

A systematic review conducted to map mHealth and mobile penetrations in sub-Saharan Africa revealed that between 2006 and 2016, 487 mHealth programs were implemented. The eastern region, which included 17 countries, and the western region, which included 16 countries, had 287 and 145 mHealth programs, respectively.[376]

mHealth emerged from telehealth, and both are made possible by modern telecommunication and information technology, which serves as a means to provide healthcare services from a distance. As noted, mHealth and telehealth can be considered subsets of eHealth.[377] This umbrella term represents the local or remote use of digital data or technology to support healthcare provision.[378]

mHealth might have started with digital epidemiology, that is, using digital traces, such as Twitter data, to assess population health in real time. One of the first famous examples of digital epidemiology was the Google Flu Trends, launched in 2008 to help predict flu epidemics and the Google search queries to track influenza-like illnesses in a population.[379]

Another earlier example of mobile tracking of infectious diseases includes Cambridge University's voluntary FluPhone app, which was developed in 2011.[380] The quest to understand how infectious diseases, such as swine flu, spread so fast[380] brought together epidemiologists, psychologists, economists, and computer scientists, and allowed the FluPhone project to work out how often people come into proximity daily. It used a mobile application on a phone to measure, comprehend, and predict how individuals change their social behaviour in response to infectious diseases.[380] According to a report by the Innovation Eye,[381] most mHealth apps are used in Europe and the United Kingdom.

mHealth and SMS in Africa

The use of short message service (SMS, a form of text messaging) in Africa began in 2004 when Ken Banks, the founder of FrontlineSMS, travelled to South Africa and Tanzania. There, he realized the usefulness of connecting communities to cheaply and easily report poaching activity on the border of the Kruger National Park by using a personal computer connected to a phone or modem, allowing users to send and receive SMS just like email.[382]

Today, FrontlineSMS provides users with software to send, manage, and receive text message interactions with communities of people, spanning the healthcare industry and election monitoring.[382] The FrontlineSMS innovation led to other relevant technologies, such as the RapidSMS tool.[383]

The RapidSMS tool was initiated in 2009 in Rwanda,[384] where community health workers were given mobile phones with a SIM (subscriber identity module) to undertake routine surveillance of health events during a woman's pregnancy, delivery, and for the first year of her child's life. By May 2010, one year after initiating the RapidSMS system, antenatal care visits in Musanze District had risen by 25%, home deliveries had declined by 54%, health facility deliveries increased by 26%, and under-five mortality had decreased by 48%.[384]

The success of RapidSMS paved the way for its scalability. USAID and the Bill and Melinda Gates Foundation purchased 10,000 and 5000 mobile phones, respectively, in support of the RapidSMS project.[384] Currently, about 45,000 community health workers and their supervisors in 475 health centres use RapidSMS, which provides information for decision making at the national level.[384] RapidSMS also formed the basis of several projects, such as mTrac, developed by UNICEF in Uganda to undertake disease surveillance and drug tracking. Other projects include Project Mwana, aimed at improving early infant diagnosis of HIV, help with postnatal follow-up and care in Zambia, and RapidSMS maternal and child health, designed to monitor pregnancy and reduce communication bottlenecks relating to maternal and childhood deaths in Rwanda.

FrontlineSMS and RapidSMS were the first few technologies in which mHealth was applied in Africa; however, there are now other prominent mHealth technologies, such as MagPi, MomConnect, GiftedMom, and Vula mobile.

Episurveyor, a mobile data collection system programmed by Datadyne, was launched in June 2009. It had more than 10,000 users in 170 countries spanning sub-Saharan Africa, Latin America, and the United

States, collecting over a million data records.[385] In January 2013, it was relaunched under the name MagPi with over 40 new features. In the health sector, MagPi is used to collect clinical patient data and public health and epidemiology information, and to track supplies and medicines for household surveys.[385] Joel Selaniko and Rose Donna founded the Datadyne company in collaboration with the Kenyan Ministry of Health after realizing that low use of mobile computers (including personal digital assistant and mobile phones) for data collection and analysis was mainly a result of the cost of available software and its complexity.

In August 2014, the National Department of Health (NDOH) implemented MomConnect as a national digital maternal health program in South Africa.[386] MomConnect was the first digital health program employing a mobile phone application to communicate with pregnant women at scale to improve their health and the health of their children. In the first year of its operation, it enrolled more than about half the number of pregnancies in the South African public sector, representing approximately half a million women.[386]

Another mHealth initiative, Vula Mobile uses the Vula Mobile Referral and Chat app to connect patients with medical practitioners so they can receive timely clinical advice and coordinated care. About 1000 referrals are made each day through the application, with about 1500 interactions between health workers. In 2020, over 120,000 patients benefited from Vula's services, and 17,000 health workers were registered on Vula Mobile, of which 7000 were active.[387]

The GiftedMom app was founded in 2015 in Cameroon to allow specialists to provide access to health information and monitoring services to pregnant women and nursing mothers.[388] The Ask A Doctor service in the GiftedMom app provides two-way SMS communication and in-app chat. The app had about 170,831 users as of December 2018.[388] The number of users and patient-doctor interactions has increased over time. In particular, the number of registered pregnant women and nursing mothers using the app increased from 300 in 2015 to 26,573 in 2016, and 84,451 in 2017.[388] In addition, the number of patient-doctor interactions through the Ask A Doctor service climbed from 300 in 2015 to 2657 in 2016, 23,768 in 2017, and 24,000 in 2018.[388]

Most of the mHealth apps in Africa, such as MomConnect and GiftedMom, focus on providing health information to mothers and collecting clinical patient data, as these tasks require mHealth for effective operation.

The scalability of the prominent mHealth technologies in Africa was highly dependent on the influx of mobile technologies on the continent, the user-friendliness of the app, and funding. Sometimes users sign up themselves or with help from health professionals. Funding allows the users to subscribe to the app for free, which increases the subscription rate. For instance, Vula Mobile won ZAR 1 million from HAVAIC, an investment firm that supports start-ups in Africa.

Some of the apps were also developed in collaboration with ministries of health in the countries, so they had political support.

Scaling Up mHealth in Africa

mHealth strategies have surged in Africa relative to other regions. According to the Global Diffusion of eHealth Survey 2015, the region of the Americas reported the highest percentage of countries with at least one mHealth program in each of the three main mHealth program categories. They are followed by the European region and then the African and Eastern Mediterranean regions.[389] Most mHealth programs were used to access or provide health services in Africa.

It is interesting to note that the percentage of countries reporting one type of mHealth program in the three main program categories (i.e., accessing/providing health services, accessing/providing health information, and collecting health information) was more than 70% in the African region.[389] Slightly over 80% of the countries in the African region employed a mHealth program related to accessing/providing health services, just under 80% adopted a program for accessing/providing health information, and above 70% undertook a program for collecting health information.[389]

In 2017, the 17 countries in the eastern region of Africa had 287 mHealth programs, while the 16 countries in the western region had 145 programs.[376] Generally, Eastern Africa is associated with more mHealth programs because of countries like Kenya, Tanzania, Malawi, and Uganda. In contrast, the northern region and countries like South Sudan, Somalia, and Rwanda are associated with low program numbers.[376] The Central African Republic also has little association with mHealth programs because the country and its neighbours lack experience with mHealth.[376]

Most countries in Africa are moderately employing mHealth strategies relative to their counterparts. South Africa has the highest potential. A study conducted by Noriega and Eveslage[390] categorized African countries based on mobile connection, use, and existence of platforms to determine their potential for success: nascent (0% to 33%), moderate (34% to 65%), and high (66% to 100%).

Rwanda, Uganda, Mozambique, and Malawi had nascent potential because of relatively low mobile connections and usage, despite having a relatively high number of platforms.[390] On the other hand, South Africa had high potential because of its strength in all three areas, while Botswana had high potential resulting from its great mobile connections and usage.[390]

Lee et al.[376] conducted a systematic review to access data on the number of mHealth programs implemented in each sub-Saharan African country between 2006 and 2016 from the WHO eHealth database, the USAID mHealth database, and the mHealth Working Group Inventory of Projects. About 487 unique mHealth programs were implemented in sub-Saharan Africa between 2006 and 2016. In particular, the authors reported that between 2006 and 2016, slightly more than 25 African countries, including Burkina Faso, Sudan, and the Democratic Republic of the Congo, had 0 to 12 mHealth programs. Seven countries, including Ethiopia, Malawi, and Zambia, had 13 to 24 programs; two countries, Ghana and South Africa, had 25 to 36 programs; Nigeria alone had 37 to 47 programs; Uganda and Tanzania had 48 to 59 programs each; and Kenya had the highest number at 60 to 71 mHealth programs.[376]

Lessons for Implementation

Lesson 1: Government Champions Can Ensure a Smooth Takeoff and Enhance Sustainability

In a qualitative study that evaluated the MomConnect program, champions were its vital enablers.[391] The involvement of South Africa's NDOH in championing the MomConnect program demonstrates how champions were critical in the sustainable and effective delivery of mHealth and telemedicine interventions.

MomConnect was one of the very few programs backed and adopted by governmental leadership because it was directly proposed and implemented by the NDOH. Engaging and building these strategic partnerships from the beginning of the implementation process can significantly support an mHealth project in adopting effective frameworks and methodologies.

Strong political will and championship from fellow project partners and the NDOH specifically made the project scale as quickly as it did. Accordingly, an implementer that was involved in the initial design of the MomConnect program stated, "[MomConnect] is regarded as a success because it had the political backing from the very beginning, and that meant it had no choice but to scale." Many donor-funded programs aim to be adopted by governmental leadership; however, few are.

The MomConnect project benefited immensely from the intense political support from the government.[391] The inability to engage most or all influential partners may adversely affect how well an mHealth initiative can take off.

The interest and advocacy from the Ministry of Health increased the motivation of the target population's involvement with the program. According to a technical person in the project focused on implementing the background information around the exchange infrastructure of the MomConnect program,

> The fact that there was buy-in, it was a ministerial project, Aaron Motsoaledi, the minister of health, was committed and basically because of that there was a lot of movement and a lot of other barriers could be gotten past, for example. The funding, there was a bit of concern about where the servers were hosted and that kind of thing. There was red tape that, I wouldn't say that was cut, but the administrative side of the red tape was accelerated because there was ministerial buy-in. What I mean by that is nothing unethical was done, but there was momentum and things didn't get bogged down on a bureaucratic level.

Champions also helped to reduce maternal and child mortality in another mHealth initiative, RapidSMS. Through the collaboration between the Korea International Cooperation Agency (KOICA) and UNICEF, the Government of Korea provided funding to scale up the RapidSMS program in Rwanda to all public health facilities. While the Rwanda Ministry of Health provided overall strategic direction and budget allocations for the RapidSMS system, UNICEF and KOICA provided funding, technical support, maintenance assistance, and capacity development.[392]

Lesson 2: Managing Costs and Accessing Funding Are Critical for Sustainability

For the MomConnect program, the high cost of data was a limitation in scaling the program, as South Africa has some of the highest data rates. In many cases, the South African market has wide ownership of mobile phones; however, the cost of setting up networks and the return for investors in mobile operators are high. For example, although discounts were obtained from telecommunication companies, they were not as good as hoped for from the national project's standpoint. The

MomConnect program found it challenging to keep costs down, with the recurring elements such as the SMS and Unstructured Supplementary Service Data (USSD) segment hampering its sustainability.

According to a consultant who supported the strategy and implementation of the NDOH's eHealth, "What was difficult on it is obviously the costs around doing this was not as, not necessarily super sustainable. The whole plan was to do it through the mobile networks and through the SMS charges, discounts were obtained, but they weren't as good as you would hope from the national project's standpoint. So trying to keep the cost down of the consumable elements, like the recurring elements, like SMS and USSD segment, keeping cost down on that was not easy, and I think there were different factors that played there that made it more difficult to really sustain it."

At scale, SMS can be very expensive and is linear in pricing; sending millions of messages a day can become costly. Donors can become uncomfortable paying these costs, because it is unsustainable in addition to being expensive. Although it was free for the user, the department was paying for those messages. According to an implementer of MomConnect, "A lot of the issues are the cost of SMS and data because we try to make the program free to the end user that's an incredible, it's a very large percentage of the program cost."

Based on worldwide mobile data pricing in 2022, the average cost of 1 GB of mobile data was determined for 233 countries. Saint Helena, located in sub-Saharan Africa, ranked 233, with the highest average cost for 1 GB of mobile data at USD 41.06.

When comparing the data for African and North American countries, 8 out of 11 countries with the most expensive mobile data rate per 1 GB are located in sub-Saharan Africa. The prices for the 8 countries start at USD 8.93 (Central African Republic) and progress from USD 9.57 (Equatorial Guinea) to USD 10.52 (Namibia), USD 12.66 (Seychelles), USD 12.94 (Togo), USD 15.55 (Botswana), USD 29.49 (São Tomé), and end at USD 41.06 (Saint Helena).

In fact, sub-Saharan Africa had 5 of the 10 most expensive countries globally. On the other hand, all North African countries experience cheaper mobile data rates than the global average of USD 3.12. However, when averaging all countries in a region, North America is the most expensive country at USD 4.98, and sub-Saharan Africa places second at USD 4.47.[393]

Regarding RapidSMS, the high financial costs associated with using technology could be a barrier to its use and expansion. The actual cost of implementing RapidSMS technology in Malawi was the cost of training community healthcare workers. The only additional operational cost was for the texts themselves, which were significantly reduced because of an agreement with the mobile providers.[394] Community health workers in Rwanda were given mobile phones to use the RapidSMS technology. The Rwandan Ministry of Health also covered the cost of the SMS.

Regarding the funding of MomConnect, one of the key partners of the project stated, "Especially when there is a reliance on donor funding, sometimes there's gaps in funding, etc. If one of those partners isn't sustained, the whole thing kind of falls over. So, getting that done is right in that sustainability model and is not unique to the program but is a challenging thing to get right."

When the Global Diffusion of eHealth Survey 2015 asked the WHO member states, particularly LMICs, to rate common barriers to mHealth program implementation by order of importance with respect to supporting universal health coverage, funding was the most important, with the majority (71%; $n = 82$) of countries rating lack of funding as an extremely important barrier.[389]

According to a technical lead in the project, "Another major challenge has been the funding. Seeing this project, it's now seen as a public good, but funders tend to only want to fund projects which are new and shiny, and exciting, and not projects which are at scale, very successful and they're working and they cost a lot of money to maintain because of the sheer size of it, and funders don't tend to want to get involved with that kind of a project. So, its been very challenging trying to get funding on an annual basis."

Lesson 3: Adaptation of the Innovation to Local Needs Engenders Acceptance and Trust

MomConnect's use of cost-efficient technology and ability to adapt to demographic characteristics, including language, literacy, and user preferences, allowed a more significant population to benefit from the technology.[391]

South Africa's high literacy rates among adults makes texting a common activity on mobile phones and, in turn, constitutes an appropriate way for mHealth programs to be scaled. A key factor in the successful operation of the MomConnect program was the language translation. The program content was translated into the 11 official languages of South Africa.

The MomConnect project used SMS, which is readily available in South Africa. To encourage usage in the context of scaling up mHealth innovations, the target population's accessibility must be known and accounted for in design and implementation.

In addition, the women were getting the service for free, and the facilities did not need to do a great deal; although it was a new system, it was not an extremely difficult one. It could be slotted into some existing processes.

According to personnel who managed the evaluation of the project, "It's to affordability, to acceptability, to accessibility, it's a lot. People like it, they like to see the information on their phone, they like the fact that it is anonymous, that they can call a helpline. They rather call the help desk in Pretoria than talk to a midwife or local nurse at their own local clinic, so to speak, it has a lot to do with the privacy or the ease of use."

We also see the importance of cost in the GiftedMom platform, which was created to provide pregnant women with follow-up services and antenatal care services via SMS. To ensure that the GiftedMom app reaches the greatest number of mothers possible, the designers ensured that the message alerts were available in several traditional languages and audio formats, allowing illiterate mothers to benefit as well.[395]

The GiftedMom smartphone app was created for both offline and online data collection and was used by community workers and medical personnel to register pregnant women and new mothers. An additional facet of GiftedMom's services is its transport system. A woman with an emergency can alert the GPS Tricycle Transport, which will pick her up and transport her to a medical facility for treatment.[396]

The app provides mapping and location information, even in rural areas, and operates without internet access using cell-tower triangulation technology.[395] The GPS technology does not require the internet to function, making it especially useful in rural areas.

Similarly, the FrontlineSMS software is simple to install and does not require an internet connection, given that many FrontlineSMS users live in remote areas where reliable internet connections are simply unavailable. FrontlineSMS was explicitly designed to serve remote communities.[397]

Lesson 4: A Good Policy Environment Reduces Regulation Barriers and Fosters Interoperability

A critical construct of the CFIR that best represents the issue of policy and regulations for mHealth is the construct of external policies and incentives, which includes policy and regulations (governmental or other central entity), external mandates, recommendations and guidelines, pay-for-performance, collaboratives, and public or benchmark reporting.[248]

An open standard framework to be shared among mHealth interventions to create an interoperable system framework is commonly used. Why? It provides a road map that incorporates the existing health technologies and systems to a scalable level to achieve a well-functioning, patient-centred electronic health information system.[398]

According to a partner involved in the initial design,

> MomConnect set out to put into practice, to take to scale the South African Normative Standards Framework, which was an actual piece of legislation that looked at how interoperability should be managed and scaled in South Africa so the technical standards to use, kind of enterprise architectures and conceptual architectures of how health programs should be managed. Essentially, MomConnect set out to show and put the framework into practice. What was easy was having those principles and standards and legislations in place already. It made it easier to get past some of the technical hurdles that might be hurdles in other places where there isn't that standard framework to start with.

In the Global Diffusion of eHealth section of the Third Global Survey report, roughly half of the countries surveyed considered the lack of legislation or regulations covering mHealth programs (51%; n = 59) as a significant barrier.[389]

The MomConnect program leveraged South Africa's Health Normative Standards Framework, which was designed to adopt an open architecture approach to serve large-scale systems development by integrating multiple applications into a single system.[386] As noted by two key informants, the use of this framework made it easier to overcome any technical hurdles that could have arisen if the framework had not been implemented from the beginning of the project. The Health Normative Standards Framework is critical for maintaining interoperability among the national health information systems,[399] and it allows mHealth programs to be implemented swiftly.[400]

Nine other African countries have also adopted digital health strategies whose titles reflect changing terminology. For example, Cameroon and Tanzania refer to them as digital health strategies. Mali, Niger, and Uganda have termed them eHealth strategies, and other countries, including the Democratic Republic of the Congo, Ethiopia, Liberia, Malawi, and Nigeria, use information/informatics or ICT strategies. Each country's strategy has a corresponding period of validity, with the shortest period at four years, such as 2020 to 2024 for Cameroon and the Democratic Republic of the Congo, and the longest period at nine years, 2020 to 2029 for Ethiopia.[401]

Introducing the policy of community health workers in Rwanda using cellular phones was strategic to meet the MDG objectives of reducing maternal and infant mortality. According to a report from Rwanda's Ministry of Health, areas in which the RapidSMS policy was implemented and well managed improved and monitored the state of health of children and mothers.[392]

The Vula app complies with the most recent Protection of Personal Information legislation, making it a more secure platform for practitioners to share patient information than other apps.[402] Using the Vula app presented a significant challenge regarding secure access to patient data and patient confidentiality. The Health Professions Council of South Africa has ethical guidelines for healthcare providers to follow when using telemedicine, but none for social media.[403]

Thus, the South African Medical Association recently released a practical and moral guide for medical professionals.[404] However, as of 2021, there was no consistent policy regarding using the Vula app.[405] A policy requiring all specialist departments to use the Vula app for referrals will significantly improve the referral process. Policy recommendations to standardize the use of the Vula app across all specialist departments and to clarify the types of referrals that best suit the Vula app would be beneficial.[405]

Summary

In light of the rapid advancement of mHealth in Africa over the last few decades, mHealth is not stalling and is spreading. However, the scalability depends on effective partnership relations, innovation costs and funding, operationalization, and policy and legislation. Partnership relations should include key participants and government champions; local adaptations must consider cost-effective technology and a sustainable funding model. mHealth initiatives must consider the literacy rate of the user base, local context, languages, the use of existing mobile technologies, comprehensibility, user attitude, acceptance, offline access, and other constraints related to the user population. Finally, country governments should continually update and establish legislation enhancing interoperability, and such frameworks should be leveraged by implementers of mHealth initiatives for more effective integration into the health system.

8
Malaria Bed Nets: A Prism of Implementation Complexity

It is now widely recognized that any attempt at malaria eradication must be a long-term commitment that involves multiple interventions, disciplines, strategies and organizations.

– Anthony Fauci

Malaria is a major global public health problem, particularly in African countries. The disease is caused by *Plasmodium* parasites, which are transmitted through the bites of infected female *Anopheles* mosquitoes.[406] Several *Anopheles* species, including *Anopheles gambiae*, *Anopheles funestus*, and *Anopheles coluzzii*, are responsible for the majority of the transmission in Africa, where the disease has the highest impact on health.[407]

In 2020, there were an estimated 241 million cases of malaria worldwide, while the estimated number of malaria deaths stood at 627,000. The WHO African Region bears a disproportionately large share of the global malaria burden. The region accounted for 95% of malaria cases and 96% of malaria deaths in 2020. Just over half of all malaria deaths worldwide occurred in four African nations: Nigeria (31.9%), the Democratic Republic of the Congo (13.2%), Tanzania (4.1%), and Mozambique (3.8%).[406] Anthony Fauci, former director of the National Institute of Allergy and Infectious Diseases at the US National Institutes of Health, captured the complexity of malaria eradication, asserting it is not a single-action task but a multifaceted approach requiring sustained effort over time and acknowledging the need for a holistic and integrated approach to overcome challenges posed by malaria.[408]

ITNs are one of the core interventions recommended for malaria control by the WHO. ITNs have decreased clinical malaria cases across

Africa. This chapter explores how malaria bed nets have been implemented in several African countries, including Tanzania, Nigeria, Uganda, and Congo, and the role that implementation science plays in leapfrogging over profound systemic and logistical challenges and navigating cultural complexities.

The use of ITNs has significantly aided in the dramatic decrease in illness and malaria-related mortality. The 2004 *Cochrane Review* "Insecticide-Treated Bed Nets and Curtains for Malaria Prevention"[51] demonstrated the efficiency of ITNs in reducing malaria prevalence, morbidity, and mortality. The review, which incorporated data from 22 randomized controlled trials, revealed that the use of ITNs reduced child mortality by 17%.[51]

In regions of consistent malaria transmission, ITNs also decreased parasite prevalence by 13%, uncomplicated malaria episodes by 50%, and severe malaria by 45%, compared with equivalent populations with no nets. In addition, findings from the *Cochrane Review* revealed that the use of ITNs reduces under-five mortality in malaria-endemic areas in sub-Saharan Africa by about a fifth.[51]

Similarly, a 2018 *Cochrane Review* conducted by Pryce et al.[409] to evaluate the impact of ITNs on malaria morbidity and mortality showed that ITNs reduce child mortality by 17% annually, which equates to saving about 6 lives annually for every 1000 children protected by ITNs.

In Mozambique, the use and scale of ITNs were estimated to have saved 14,040 lives of children under age five from 2012 to 2018.[410] An evaluation of a social marketing program implemented in Tanzania in May 1997 to scale up the use of ITNs confirms that ITNs have a substantial impact on morbidity and malaria mortality. The study's findings show that the prevalence of anemia in the study group (those who owned ITNs) fell from 49% to 26% and that ITNs had a protective efficacy of 62% and 63% on parasitemia and anemia prevalence, respectively.[411]

How did such an impactful innovation come to be?

According to Steve Lindsay and Mary Gibson's historical perspective on bed net development, bed nets were initially used as a defence against blood-sucking insects. However, treated and untreated bed nets were exceedingly rare until the middle of the 1940s. The use of bed nets was first documented in the Middle East around the sixth century BCE,[412] and they were made of flax, although hemp and palm fibres were sometimes used.[413]

In pre-colonial times, diverse ethnic groups made use of bed nets. For example, the Fulani and Hausa people of West Africa slept beneath thin grass mats with a net pattern. Although the Fulani viewed them as protection against evil spirits, the Mandinka used them for privacy and protection against mosquitoes.[414] Lindsay and Gibson believe that bed nets were developed independently because their use has been observed in isolated populations scattered in different parts of the world. During World War II, American and German forces employed ITNs to protect their troops from vector-borne illnesses, including malaria and leishmaniasis.[412] Malaria prevention changed dramatically following World War II, when insecticide-based methods were first widely applied against adult mosquitoes.

The most important development at the time was the introduction of DDT (dichloro-diphenyl-trichloroethane) insecticide, which quickly became the primary weapon.[415,416] During this period, bed nets and jungle hammocks were also treated with insecticides to protect soldiers and citizens from malaria and other insect-borne diseases in Southeast Asia.[417] An experimental assessment of the durability of synthetic pyrethroids impregnated in various fabrics for the production of mosquito nets was documented by Hervy and Sales in 1980.

A few years later, information from West Africa suggests a group under the direction of the French scientist Pierre Carnevale may have invented the modern ITN for mosquito control; they were the first to test ITNs in controlled experiments inside huts in Bobo-Dioulasso, Burkina Faso. The trial results show that insecticide (permethrin) treated nets reduced the number of *An. gambiae* and *An. funestus* mosquitoes entering the experimental huts by 70%. The trial established that even though permethrin-treated nets do not entirely isolate humans from Anopheles mosquitoes they significantly reduce human-vector contact to approximately 70%.[418] Use of mosquito nets for malaria prevention was not widespread until the late 1980s and early 1990s, two decades after the initial attempt at a global campaign to eradicate malaria, which had primarily depended on IRS (indoor residual spray) with DDT.[414]

As the public health emphasis shifted back to prevention, with a revived role for vector control (in accordance with the 1978 Alma Ata declaration), ITNs were officially included in the worldwide malaria control policy.[419] Roll Back Malaria (RBM), founded in 1998, became a key proponent of increased use of ITNs.

The operational use of ITNs by national malaria control programs, particularly in Africa, encountered the need to treat the mosquito nets once every six months or after two or three washings. To address this issue, long-lasting insecticide nets (LLINs) were produced. LLINs are nets treated in the factory with an insecticide incorporated into the net fabric, which makes the insecticide last at least 20 washes in standard laboratory testing and three years of recommended use under field conditions. With LLINs, the time-consuming method of re-treating old nets is no longer necessary.[420]

Scaling Up Malaria Bed Nets

Africa has the world's highest malaria burden, driven by favourable environmental conditions and the presence of the most virulent parasite species, *Plasmodium falciparum* and *Anopheles* mosquitoes, which have a "strong human-biting habit."[421] While sub-Saharan Africa bears the greatest impact from the disease, West African countries are especially vulnerable to malaria because of extreme poverty and a lack of access to care.[421] The scale-up of ITN use in Africa is paramount to reducing the mortality and morbidity of malaria.

Mosquito net (ITNs) use is one of the core malaria interventions in Africa, particularly for pregnant women and children under the age of five. Following the Abuja Declaration by African heads of state in 2000, the adoption of ITNs in Africa increased steadily, but the proportion of children under five and expecting women using mosquito nets was still relatively low by 2003. Between 1999 and 2004, national representative household surveys provided the first coverage estimates for 36 sub-Saharan African nations. Only 3% of children under the age of five and 2.8% of pregnant women who participated in these studies slept with ITNs.[423] These unacceptably low coverage estimates were partly explained by the low availability of nets in African households, with just 18% of households having one or more mosquito nets.[422,423]

However, since 2004, there has been a significant increase in the adoption of ITN usage and ownership in African countries, thanks to the funding opportunities available, the support from international organizations for the mass distribution of ITNs, and cutting-edge delivery strategies, like social marketing. For instance, a survey conducted in Niger before the 2005/2006 nationwide mass campaign showed the percentage of ITNs owned by all households was only 6.3%; following the campaign, the percentage of ITNs owned rapidly increased to 65.1%.[424]

A morbidity survey carried out in Togo in September 2004 revealed that just 0.4% of children under the age of five slept under an ITN the night before the survey. However, in December 2004, the country conducted its first nationwide distribution of ITNs for the prevention of malaria. After the campaign, household ownership of ITNs increased from 8.0% to 62.5%. Also, 43.5% of children under the age of five slept under an ITN the night before the follow-up survey.[425]

In 2017, a total of 220 million ITNs were distributed worldwide, of which 175 million (81% of the total distributed ITNs) were distributed across sub-Saharan Africa. The percentage of households in sub-Saharan Africa with at least one ITN increased from 47% in 2010 to 72% in 2017.[426]

The burden of malaria in the world is disproportionately severe in the African region. As noted, according to a WHO report, the high prevalence of malaria in Africa is primarily due to the long lifespan and the strong human-biting habit of the African species (*Anopheles gambiae*) that transmits malaria.[427] As of 2020, over half of all malaria deaths worldwide occurred in just four African nations: Nigeria, Congo, Tanzania, and Mozambique.[406] To increase the use of malaria bed nets in Africa, the governments of African nations have worked in partnership with international organizations over the years. As far back as 1998, the RBM initiative was launched by the WHO, the World Bank, UNICEF, and United Nations Development Programme.[428]

In 2000, African heads of state endorsed the initiative at a summit in Abuja.[429] With the goal established by African heads of state to protect 60% of all pregnant women and children by 2005, the widespread implementation of ITNs was one of the strategies adopted by the initiative to reduce malaria morbidity and death.[430] Since the RBM initiative's endorsement, large-scale programs have been implemented in African countries to increase the use of ITNs.

For instance, in Tanzania, through a public-private partnership known as the Tanzanian National Voucher Scheme (TNVS), a subsidy program was created in 2004 to provide LLINs to pregnant women and children under the age of five. By subsidizing the costs of ITNs, this program has expanded the availability and accessibility of ITNs to pregnant women and infants.[431] In addition, from 2008 to 2010, a mass distribution campaign of LLINs was carried out in Tanzania, with 9 million LLINs being supplied free to children under the age of five on Tanzania's mainland.[432]

Furthermore, in 2010 and 2011, a universal coverage campaign funded by the Global Fund to Fight AIDS, Tuberculosis, and Malaria, and led by the Ministry of Health and Social Welfare, was implemented in the country to distribute LLINs to areas and regions not yet reached by previous initiatives.[420]

Although Nigeria is currently the country with the highest burden of malaria, a commendable effort has been made by the Nigerian government and international organizations in the past decade. The Nigerian government, at various levels of governance, has embarked on the free distribution of ITNs to caregivers of children under the age of five.[433]

A survey conducted in Nigeria between 2000 and 2004 shows that four years after ITNs were introduced to the public, awareness of ITNs increased from 7% to 60%.[434] The National Malaria Control Strategic Plan (2014–20) reports show that from 2009 to 2013, about 58 million LLINs were distributed as part of the universal LLIN campaigns to protect an estimated 29 million households from malaria. LLINs had been delivered in 14 of Nigeria's 36 states by August 2010.[435] The partnered organizations responsible for LLINs distribution include the World Bank in seven states (Akwa-Ibom, Anambra, Bauchi, Gombe, Jigawa, Kano, and Rivers), the Global Fund in three states (Niger, Ogun, and Ekiti), and UNICEF in four states (Adamawa, Sokoto, Kaduna, and Kebbi).[436,437]

NetMark, a 10-year, USD 65.4 million USAID-funded initiative aimed at lowering the burden of malaria in sub-Saharan Africa by improving commercial supply and public demand for ITNs, collaborated with a community project in Nasarawa state to implement a targeted subsidy scheme in seven local government areas (LGAs). This program boosted under-five ownership and usage of ITNs within the seven LGAs. In addition, NetMark distributed 673,000 LLINs donated by USAID and the Canadian government to 18 LGAs in Cross River State in 2005.[437] Additionally, in February 2022, the government of Nasarawa State collaborated with the United States President's Malaria Initiative to deliver approximately 2 million ITNs in Lafia, the state capital.[438]

Implementation Strategies

Designing for Improved Adoption

One of the main documented reasons for mosquito net non-usage and inconsistent use is discomfort.[439,440,441] According to Pulford et al.,[441] education or behavioural change strategies would not affect the physical features of the mosquito nets that cause discomfort. Thus, modification of mosquito net design is paramount.

Human-centred design research was carried out in 2017 by Johns Hopkins Center for Communication Programs (CCP) researchers to determine the type of mosquito nets Ghanaians wanted.[440] Human-centred design is a creative problem-solving strategy involving working directly with key interested groups to gain insights vital to developing valuable products for a certain market or audience.

Though LLINs were available through free distribution channels in Ghana, most study participants reported the nets were inconvenient, uncomfortable, and unattractive, rendering them undesirable for use.

The study participants described the process of hanging and entering and exiting the LLIN as challenging and stressful. The LLIN's polyethylene material was also criticized by some as being "hard" and "rough" to the touch, and several people voiced worries about the pesticide treatment and potential adverse effects of its use (e.g., burning sensation in the eyes or on the skin). Participants also talked about how LLINs didn't match their ideal bedroom and home decor in terms of aesthetics.[440]

The CCP researchers argued that for LLIN use to increase among Ghanaians, the design of LLINs had to change. The new designs had to be convenient, comfortable, and attractive while still protecting against mosquito bites. To address these concerns, the researchers designed and tested various LLIN attributes, focusing on a more convenient way to hang the net, a more attractive silhouette, and a zipper to allow the user to enter and exit with ease while still ensuring a sealed, mosquito-free zone. Consumer views and preliminary ideas for new design features were shared with manufacturers worldwide to produce LLINs in Ghana.[440] If this net design is successful, it could encourage the middle class to use LLINs more frequently and to buy LLINs.

In May 2019, one of the CCP researchers visited Ghana to examine the new designed and manufactured nets. Two of the new designs that were already available for sale were a conical net with a zippered entry and a pop-up tent net. According to a CCP researcher report, Ghanaians were willing and excited to buy the newly designed net.[442]

The target population's willingness to pay for LLINs with the recommended features was captured in a separate discrete choice experiment, which validated the desirability of these attributes.[443]

To develop successful policies, human-centred approaches for increasing bed net usage should closely align with increased comfort and personal lifestyles, which are critical when designing bed nets. Heat is a commonly cited barrier to bed net usage and contributes to the low reported use.[444,445] One policy consideration would be to give residents information on ways to reduce heat in sleeping spaces, which could include using light bulbs that emit less heat and lighter-coloured curtains to trap less heat overnight.[439]

Nets could be manufactured using white material (polyethylene, polyester, etc.) to trap less heat than dark nets do. Discomfort from rigid material (i.e., nylon) was also cited as a reason people refrain from using bed nets.[439] Using softer material (e.g., polyethylene) will help curb the use of these nets for unintended purposes (e.g., using the nets as window curtains). Standardized (one-size-fits-all) approaches to reduce malaria transmission levels are insufficient when trying to eliminate malaria nationwide. Areas with widespread resistance to insecticides should be considered when tailoring the distribution of nets based on resistance profiles.

Installation difficulties are a common reason cited for not using ITNs regularly.[446] Materials and tools for hanging the nets (i.e., hooks and clips) should be distributed with the bed nets to ease the installation process, along with conducting campaigns on how to install these nets, within a month of distribution.[447]

To increase consistent use of bed nets, portable nets (i.e., pop-up/self-supporting nets) should be provided whenever necessary to reduce difficulties in assembly for specific groups, such as children and pregnant women. This design was proposed by Pulford et al.[441] because of the need for external supporting structures and constant difficulties associated with hanging nets in specific households.

Accounting for Cost in Implementation

According to research, a significant obstacle to ITN ownership is cost.[445,448,449,450,451] The increasing availability of nets among the poorest rural populations may not result in increased net use until the cost of nets is no longer a barrier. Guyatt et al.[452] emphasized that other approaches, such as free distribution and subsidized pricing for ITNs, need to be considered because poverty is pervasive among the rural communities most at risk for malaria.

Since the WHO's recommendation of ITNs for malaria prevention, many African nations have adopted policies of free mass distribution of ITNs, especially for rural communities that might not have the financial means to purchase ITNs. For instance, between 2004 and 2015, Kenyans, particularly those in rural areas, received roughly 50.2 million free ITNs.[453] As part of the universal LLIN campaigns, over 58 million LLINs were distributed between 2009 and 2013 to protect an estimated 29 million households from malaria.[435] In 2014, a nationwide free mass distribution campaign in Zambia distributed 6 million LLINs in 6 of 10 regions in 4 months, between June and September.[454]

The Tanzanian government implemented the TNVS in 2004. Between 2004 and 2014, the Scheme provided highly subsidized ITNs to pregnant women and newborns. A printed voucher with a face value of TZS 2750 (USD 2.75 in 2004) was provided to every pregnant woman who visited a prenatal clinic. The woman then paid between USD 0.5 and USD 1.5 to purchase an ITN (current retail prices: USD 3.0 to USD 4.0). An assessment of the intervention showed that between 2005 and 2007, ITN coverage for infants increased from 16% to 34% and for pregnant women from 11% to 23%.[455] Aside from the TNVS, all taxes (VAT) on nets and netting materials were abolished by the end of 2004. According to Magesa et al.,[456] the removal of all taxes on nets and netting materials resulted in a considerable decline in retail prices. The demand for ITN increased significantly because of the lower price.

In 2004, a voucher scheme was implemented in the Volta region of Ghana as a sustainable delivery strategy for increasing the use of ITNs. Pregnant women who visited a prenatal clinic received a voucher for GHS 40,000 (USD 4.20). The woman took the voucher to an authorized store that sells ITNs, paid the necessary top-up amount, and turned in the voucher.[457] As a result of the voucher scheme program, ownership of mosquito nets increased from 38.3% to 45.4%.[458]

There is a need for governing bodies and policymakers to continue working on finding appropriate finance- and income-targeted strategies to improve use and access to nets, especially by those living in poverty, who often bear a higher burden of cases than their wealthier counterparts. Accordingly, household-level incentives, such as providing a redeemable coupon for a bed net, have been found to significantly increase the immediate use of ITNs in target households in Madagascar.[459] Providing incentives to promote behaviour change is a tool that can be used to increase the effectiveness of distribution programs and sustainability of bed net usage, especially in the short term; bed net use was substantially higher in the intervention group (99% versus 78%).[459]

To finance the distribution of bed nets where the malaria burden is high and to ensure the nets reach the populations equitably, region-specific data and background information are needed ahead of distribution. This is particularly important for women with maternal anemia and in areas in which there is very low access to resources and health facilities.[460] To mitigate these effects, during their antenatal clinic visits, pregnant women should be educated on the consequences of not using bed nets and given resources, such as instruction pamphlets and bed net incentives.

Strategizing for Implementation in Rural or Distant Communities

Malaria is an example of a disease for which the risk differs between rural and urban settings.[461] Studies have shown that malaria incidence is generally lower in urban areas than in rural areas.[462,463] Poor socioeconomic conditions and suitable *Anopheles* mosquitoes breeding sites contribute to the high prevalence of malaria in rural areas.[464,465] However, it is worth noting that slums in urban settings are just as vulnerable as rural areas, given their poor sanitary conditions.

Multifaceted approaches to promoting bed net usage are required to combat the different caseloads of malaria in urban communities and in rural/distant communities that have lower access to major transport links and health facilities. There are consistent inequities between urban and rural populations in terms of bed net delivery, indicative of alarmingly more inadequate bed net coverage in rural and poor populations.[466,467] A potential solution is to shift the focus towards increasing the number of distribution points closer to rural locations in the Democratic Republic of the Congo. Particularly in places with increased poverty levels and fewer resources, people are more likely to allocate their financial and other resources in ways they deem to be of immediate need and essential to life (i.e., using free bed nets for other purposes they believe are more important). Governments and policymakers must clarify that bed nets prevent malaria and emphasize the direct benefit of averting hospital stays and costs during infection and after release. Distribution programs may increase initial ITN coverage, but to maintain its sustainability after distribution and gaining population trust, collaboration between community members and community leaders is necessary.

Distance and accessibility to ITN distribution stations are significant barriers to ownership, as access to distribution points remains limited in many rural communities. The possibility of purchasing an ITN is directly proportional to the distance from an ITN distribution location.[468] Chuma et al.[469] conducted a study to identify and address barriers to access and use of ITNs among Kenya's poorest populations. It revealed that bad roads were a significant barrier to accessing ITNs in rural communities.

Therefore, improving infrastructure may make producers or wholesalers more eager to provide ITNs to merchants and healthcare facilities. As a result of improved infrastructure, manufacturers and wholesalers may be more likely to deliver ITNs to retailers and healthcare facilities in remote areas. Particularly in rural communities, health professionals can supply ITNs during routine outreach programs, and community members can more easily travel to outreach and market centres if ITNs are readily available.

Control program managers can design ways to incorporate community-based distribution of ITNs into existing distribution strategies to move large numbers of ITNs into rural areas.[470] Community-based distribution here refers to selecting and training local community members to work as community-based distributors of ITNs. ITN distribution promoters, such as the officials of the state and local governments' malaria control programs and other non-governmental ITN promoters, might recruit community-based distributors alongside community leaders and train them. The community-based distributors will obtain ITNs regularly from both public and non-governmental sources and sell them to their community members.[470]

To ensure the sustainability of community-based distribution, community-based distributors could be given a stipend. Between 1992 and 2002, the African Medical and Research Foundation used a community-based approach to deliver ITNs to Sagana, a rural community in Kenya consisting of five villages. The strategy depended on organized community groups recruited by the foundation to promote ITNs. The groups sold ITNs to householders, resulting in a 34% increase in ITN ownership.[451]

Addressing Misconceptions Head On

Awareness of bed net usage and its positive attributes is essential for increasing bed net adoption, particularly by combatting misconceptions about malaria and bed nets. Accordingly, health literacy rates and directed health education or promotion efforts must be addressed.

In Africa, people have some potentially harmful misconceptions concerning ITNs, and the misuse of ITNs has been reported. Some people view ITNs as an inconvenience that offers only mediocre protection against a minor sickness. Reports have shown that ITNs have been used as wedding veils in Tanzania and Uganda, used for fishing in Kenya and Zambia, and used to preserve plants and crops in Sierra Leone.[471] Education and awareness on proper ITN use are important to correct any misunderstanding and misuse of bed nets.

A quasi-experimental study was conducted in a rural area of Nigeria's Ogun State (Ijebu North local government area) to investigate the impact of health education on ITN usage. The study consisted of a structured educational program with a curriculum adapted from the national malaria control program. The study's findings confirm that health education significantly increased the use of ITNs.[472] If ITNs are made available and are accompanied by health education intervention, the adoption of ITNs should greatly increase in rural regions.

The mass distribution campaign to encourage community members to accept and use ITNs in Zambia in 2014 included a promotion educational activity using several means, such as personal interactions, mass media, and print media. The national Information, Education, and Communication Technical Working Group team of specialists created key messages to ensure quality, harmonization, and collaboration.[454] This team created an information, education, and communication package that included radio guides, radio station scripts, and brochures for ITNs. Materials such as pamphlets and fliers were used to inform the public about the campaign and the importance of long-term ITN use.

It was discovered that radio broadcasts of important ITN messages allowed for valuable interaction between communities and health workers. The radio broadcasts were created in English and local languages, which the communities appreciated.[454] The creation of key messages for information dissemination and the method of dissemination through interpersonal communication, mass media, and print media, along with practical teaching to households on net hanging and maintenance, increased community knowledge and uptake of the malaria intervention.

As evidence of the impact of household awareness-raising efforts, 91% of women ages 15 to 59 reported using mosquito nets as a malaria prevention technique in 2015, compared with 80% in 2013–14.[454]

I propose the use of peer education, where students learn from other students to promote bed net usage, and in-school behaviour change education strategies to raise awareness through school activities (i.e., assemblies in which students would be involved in disseminating action areas among school staff and students). Developing a mobile educational program, mainly targeted at parents, that travels from community to community would help tackle misconceptions (e.g., the association of bed nets with infertility).[473] Group sessions or meetings and community-wide campaigns using global volunteers from non-profit organizations and NGOs can be used to discuss concerns over the use of bed nets and to note any considerations for future design or distribution of nets. Messages and posters can be sent home to ensure that populations are following the public health measures (i.e., properly hanging bed nets and taking medications, and describing what malaria is). Schools could also serve as centres for distributing bed nets.

Additional research using household surveys should be done to better understand user preferences, usage patterns across the country, and alternative uses of these nets. By collecting data on personal preferences and cultural- or community-level beliefs, campaigns can tailor bed nets to meet the population's needs and increase their acceptability while also refuting any misconceptions. Local telecommunication platforms (e.g., radios and television) can be used to disseminate health messages related to malaria and bed net usage and to promote positive behaviour change. This will include the support of local radio stations, particularly those in rural areas that answer to the informational needs of marginalized populations (i.e., producing content in local languages).

Health promotion efforts in Ethiopia have designed interactive strategies in rural communities to help mitigate the adverse effects of malaria through roadshows that address behavioural challenges, such as misconceptions on malaria prevention and treatment. Ultimately, these roadshows were shown to significantly increase bed net usage levels among attendees and their knowledge of malaria, its prevention methods, and its consequences.[474]

Planning in Advance for Distribution Programs

ITNs mass distribution strategies differ by country, with each country having its own goals and challenges. With the transition to universal coverage, ITN distribution campaigns have increased in size and complexity, making early and coordinated planning crucial. Good planning is essential to the success of any mass distribution campaign, whether stand-alone or integrated, national or subnational, or universal coverage.

The 2014 mass campaign, which distributed 6 million LLINs, was the largest nationwide LLIN distribution in Zambia, compared with 235,800 LLINs distributed in 2008 and 2.9 million LLINs distributed on a rolling basis in 2013.[454] The success of this campaign was due to the intense planning carried out before the implementation phase. The timely and thorough micro-planning at the national and subnational levels made it possible to estimate the need for LLINs with accuracy and efficiency, which was necessary to execute the mass campaign.

The Zambian Ministry of Health and its collaborators created a thorough micro-plan for the 2014 mass distribution. The micro-plan detailed the general needs, the procurement plans, and the roles and duties of the national (central), province, and district levels to guide the mass campaign.[454] The mass distribution plan was communicated to communities (including local chiefs and traditional leaders) six months in advance. This early notification meant community chiefs, leaders, and volunteers could adequately plan and orient themselves in their catchment areas, which promoted program ownership. Additionally, several workshops with provincial and district planners and district malaria focal points were arranged to ensure that each province or district knew the scope of the logistics required to carry out the mass distribution.[454] Following the mass campaigns, a national malaria survey revealed significant improvements in LLIN ownership in Zambia, with 77% of households owning at least one ITN.[475]

In a recent systematic review on the barriers to and facilitators of malaria bed nets in Tanzania, the results highlighted that one vital area in the development of successful implementation was detailed planning for the execution of ITN distribution programs.[448]

The results showed that adequate planning before net distribution could lead to a more successful implementation of ITNs in Tanzania. This included selecting the proper strategies for promoting and distributing ITNs, which remain essential steps.

In Tanzania, the National Malaria Control Program and the Zanzibar Malaria Elimination Program led LLIN implementation efforts in mainland Tanzania and Zanzibar. Their established distribution programs have been remarkable successes, such as the Tanzania National Voucher Scheme and the Under-Five Catch-Up Campaign.

A unique distribution method is direct net transactions, in which ITNs are sold the same day as distribution. This method guarantees a net immediately after purchase, strengthening the trust in the implementation project and the product itself.

The planning of strategies to be used during implementation is necessary to ensure the highest coverage possible. The planning and strategy for net distribution correspond to the *process* domain of the CFIR.[248] This determinant framework comprises five broad domains and 39 constructs that guide the systematic assessment of factors that influence the intervention's implementation. The most prominent CFIR domains related to malaria bed nets implementation in Africa are intervention adaptation, individuals, and processes.

Conclusion

Malaria remains the principal cause of mortality and morbidity in Africa. The ultimate goal of current malaria control strategies is to reduce its transmission level and mortality. Malaria bed nets, an evidenced-based innovation, have a demonstrated impact on saving and improving African lives. Overall, bed net usage has a significant effect on malaria mortality. Despite recent advances in scaling up malaria bed nets, implementation challenges remain for several reasons, such as cost, optimal design, difficulty in reaching rural communities, misconceptions, and complexities in planning. By systematically accounting for these factors, implementation scientists and partners are designing strategies that allowed the adoption, spread, and use of bed nets to continue flourishing.

9

Polio Eradication: Are We There Yet?

Polio's pretty special because once you get an eradication, you no longer have to spend money on it; it's just there as a gift for the rest of time.

– Bill Gates

In August 2020, the African region was declared free of wild polio, a significant achievement for the global polio eradication effort. However, in 2022, wild poliovirus was detected in Africa again. Since then, the region has been grappling with increasing cases of the polio variant.

This chapter explores the history of the poliovirus in Africa, its epidemiological patterns, and its societal implications. It also examines the transformative role and impact of polio vaccines in Africa, emphasizing milestones, successes, and challenges.

The world has come a long way in its fight for polio eradication. Successful eradication means children will no longer suffer the devastating consequences of this disease. In an interview in 2013, Bill Gates spoke on the ongoing financial and health benefits of eradicating polio. Investing in polio eradication efforts has an immediate effect on the health threat posed by disease while also eliminating related costs and freeing up resources for other health priorities.[476]

In 1988, the WHO partnered with Rotary International, the CDC, and several national governments to launch the Global Polio Eradication Initiative (GPEI). The goal of this initiative was to eradicate the poliovirus globally. Before the GPEI began, polio was wreaking havoc in 125 countries, with 350,000 children infected worldwide. Unrelenting efforts reduced that number to only 6 cases by 2021.

However, polio seems to be making a comeback. Identification and treatment of the virus still pose challenges because of persistent barriers that must be overcome to achieve complete eradication. Although the GPEI has done an exemplary job, clear challenges still threaten the viability of the eradication program.

Polio was first formally recognized as a condition in 1840 by German physician Jakob Heine. Before the existence of a vaccine, those who survived the disease lived with lifelong consequences, such as limb malformations and permanent breathing complications.[477] Polio outbreaks continued to grow, and in the United States in the late 1940s, an average of 35,000 people each year were contracting polio.[478]

There are two types of polio vaccines. The inactive poliovirus vaccine (IPV) is given as an injection into the leg or arm. This vaccine is produced from wild-type strains of poliovirus that are inactivated with formalin. The oral poliovirus vaccine (OPV) is taken by mouth.[479] The OPV is made up of a mixture of live attenuated strains derived from three different serotypes. Although the OPV is no longer administered in the United States, it is still used in other parts of the world.[480]

The first efforts to find a cure for polio began in 1935, when British American virologist Maurice Brodie attempted to develop a vaccine using formalin and experimented with it using 20 monkeys and 3000 children with little success.[481] However, research into polio vaccine development was continued by other scientists. American virologist Jonas Salk created the first successful IPV by incubating the virus in monkey kidney cells and inactivating it with formalin. By 1954, the IPV was being tested through a placebo-controlled study in which 1.6 million children in Canada, Finland, and the United States were enrolled. The immunogenicity of this vaccine, which was adopted throughout the United States in 1955, decreased within a few years of vaccination, and it was difficult to mass produce the vaccine because of the large number of monkeys required. This led to a change in the manufacturing process in 1980 that concentrated and purified the polio antigens, leading to an increase in vaccine immunogenicity.[482]

In 1960, Dr. Albert Sabin developed a trivalent oral vaccine based on a trial of 26,033 children from a city of 100,000 in South America. This OPV was selected for licensing from 1961 to 1963 for widespread application in the United States. By 1962, the first nationwide poliomyelitis vaccination campaign was launched in Cuba.[482]

The use of an OPV was considered powerful when eliminating polio was the goal, as it was able to interrupt the chain of transmission, in contrast to IPV, which could not stop transmission between children.[477] With increased traction of the polio vaccine and increased assistance from the WHO, large-scale global projects started taking place. In 1979, Rotary International, a non-profit organization, began a project

Figure 9.1. Milestones in Global Polio Vaccination Efforts

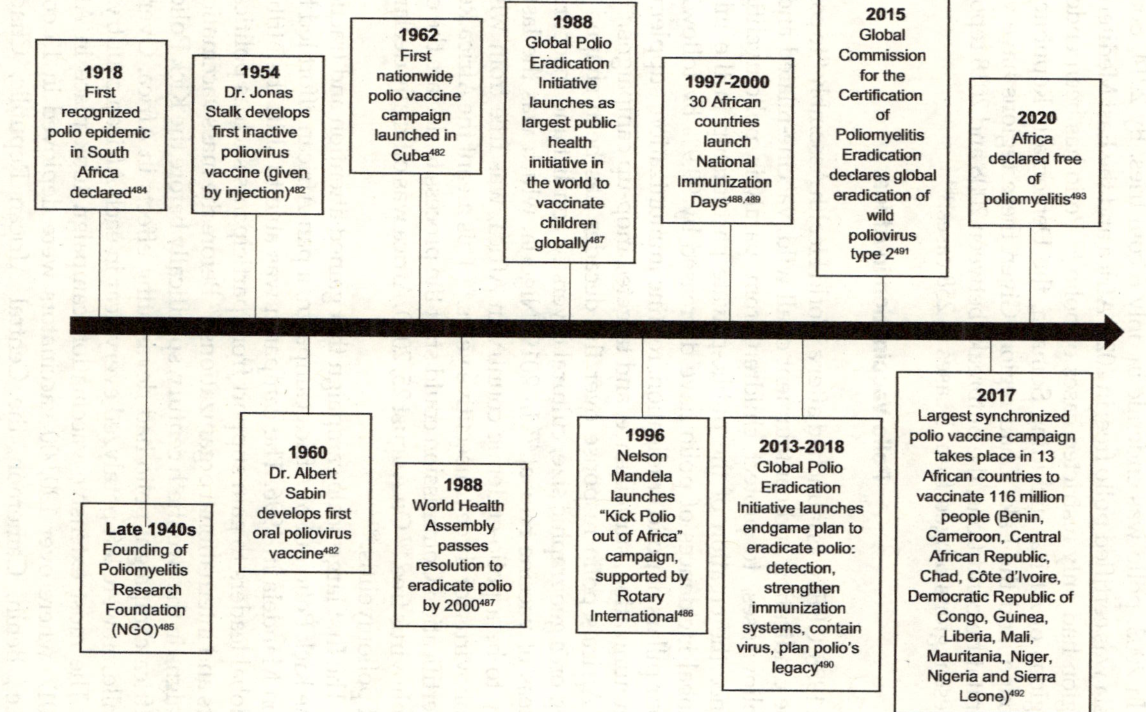

1918 First recognized polio epidemic in South Africa declared[484]
Late 1940s Founding of Poliomyelitis Research Foundation (NGO)[485]
1954 Dr. Jonas Stalk develops first inactive poliovirus vaccine (given by injection)[482]
1960 Dr. Albert Sabin develops first oral poliovirus vaccine[482]
1962 First nationwide polio vaccine campaign launched in Cuba[482]
1988 World Health Assembly passes resolution to eradicate polio by 2000[487]
1988 Global Polio Eradication Initiative launches as largest public health initiative in the world to vaccinate children globally[487]
1996 Nelson Mandela launches "Kick Polio out of Africa" campaign, supported by Rotary International[486]
1997-2000 30 African countries launch National Immunization Days[488,489]
2013-2018 Global Polio Eradication Initiative launches endgame plan to eradicate polio: detection, strengthen immunization systems, contain virus, plan polio's legacy[490]
2015 Global Commission for the Certification of Poliomyelitis Eradication declares global eradication of wild poliovirus type 2[491]
2017 Largest synchronized polio vaccine campaign takes place in 13 African countries to vaccinate 116 million people (Benin, Cameroon, Central African Republic, Chad, Côte d'Ivoire, Democratic Republic of Congo, Guinea, Liberia, Mali, Mauritania, Niger, Nigeria and Sierra Leone)[492]
2020 Africa declared free of poliomyelitis[493]

to vaccinate 6 million children in the Philippines over multiple years, and other mass vaccination campaigns were run in 1995 in China and India.[477]

In 2003, polio was endemic in only 6 countries. By 2014, Southeast Asia was certified polio free; in 2020, Africa and the East Mediterranean region had only restricted cases of polio.[477] Polio has been endemic to regions of Africa, including Somalia, the Democratic Republic of the Congo, and the Lake Chad region. Given these regions have varying sanitation conditions, the outbreaks between 2008 and 2018 reported in these regions ranged from 3 cases to 258 cases.[483]

Polio Vaccination in Africa

In 1988, GPEI was launched after a World Health Assembly "to complete the eradication and containment of all wild, vaccine-related and Sabin polioviruses, to protect children from paralytic poliomyelitis."[494,495] Since the creation of the public-private partnership in the initiative, global incidences of polio have decreased by 99.9% by following the four pillars of polio eradication: routine immunization, supplementary immunization, surveillance, and targeted mop-up campaigns.[496]

Africa's polio response over the decades has been shaped by the region's geographic size, cultural diversity, conflict and insecurity, and areas of vaccine refusal.[477] In 2019, Nigeria, which was the last country to be a polio-endemic country in Africa, was free from wild-type poliovirus for three consecutive years.[497] This meant the Africa Regional Certification Commission could start the process to declare the country poliovirus free.[497] On August 25, 2020, Africa was officially declared free of poliomyelitis.[493]

The first large-scale campaign that gained attention and traction was the Kick Polio out of Africa campaign, a pan-African effort led by Nelson Mandela in 1996. The campaign was able to shift the attitudes of global leaders to gain support from participants such as political leaders and international organizations.[492] Before the mass vaccination campaigns in the twentieth century, specifically before the Kick Polio out of Africa campaign, polio had devastating effects in Africa. Over 75,000 children were left paralyzed every year in each African country.[492]

The most extensive vaccination campaign took place in Africa in 2017, where over 190,000 vaccinators were deployed in 13 countries (i.e., Benin, Cameroon, the Central African Republic, Chad, Côte d'Ivoire, the Democratic Republic of the Congo, Guinea, Liberia, Mali, Mauritania, Niger, Nigeria, and Sierra Leone) to vaccinate over 116 million children over one week.[492] The OPV was selected and administered through an enormous coordinated effort by healthcare workers and volunteers, who worked 12 hours per day and travelled into remote villages through difficult physical terrain.[492]

Impact of Polio Vaccines in Africa

A key player in the polio vaccination efforts in Africa has been the GPEI. The GPEI is a public-private partnership led by national governments with six partners: the WHO, Rotary International, the CDC, UNICEF, the Bill and Melinda Gates Foundation, and Global Alliance for Vaccine Initiatives (GAVI). The initiative was successful in working with 200 countries and 20 million volunteers, vaccinating over 2.5 billion children thus far, and receiving a USD 17 billion international investment.[495]

Another key player is the Global Polio Laboratory Network (coordinated by the WHO), which is deeply integrated with field case-based surveillance to provide information for programmatic and immunization activities.[498] It was established in 1990 to distinguish cases of acute flaccid paralysis (AFP) caused by poliovirus from those caused by other diseases.[499]

This network includes 146 WHO-accredited polio laboratories in 92 countries across the six WHO regions of the world. The network is staffed with virologists, epidemiologists, clinicians, and national immunization program staff, backed by the laboratories, to carry out effective polio surveillance. Effective surveillance begins with standardized protocols, isolating the virus, identifying and screening for the virus, and conducting genome sequencing of the virus.[499]

Achieving the goals of the GPEI in Africa was aided by the Global Polio Laboratory Network.[493] Several studies have emerged that validated the contribution of the African polio laboratories and their scientific evidence, including early detection of wild-type strain outbreaks, polio diagnostics, and next-generation sequencing to study polio's molecular epidemiology.[498,500-502] This network has been critical in eradicating polio in Africa, providing timely and accurate data to the GPEI to assist in vaccination efforts.[498]

The main pillars identified to have a critical impact on the mortality and morbidity caused by poliomyelitis in Africa include high infant routine immunization coverage, regular supplemental immunization, and active case-based surveillance of cases in children younger than 15 years old.[493] For example, a 13-year analysis of polio vaccine campaigns in Guinea-Bissau found that mortality rate ratios of children between ages 1 and 3 years were lower after OPV campaigns, indicating an association between OPV campaigns and decreased child mortality.[503] A combination of these strategies led to a reduction of wild-type cases by 99%,[504] with Nigeria the last remaining endemic area until 2020.[493]

Mobilizing domestic financial resources to contribute to polio outbreak response efforts by the WHO and the GPEI was essential to polio eradication. The GPEI reported that the initiative's immunization campaigns successfully reached 40 million children across 20 countries in Africa.[505]

Critical Factors for Polio Eradication

1. Anticipate and Deal with Fears and Rumours Head On

Fears and rumours have always been significant factors in polio eradication in Africa. Fears are usually associated with rumours, suspicions, and past experiences with other diseases, rendering parents and caregivers reluctant to take up polio programs.

Before Africa was declared free of wild polio in August 2020, several stories hampered polio vaccination. For example, in Nigeria, a fatwa (a legal ruling on Islamic law given by a qualified scholar) was issued in 2003 that the polio vaccine was intended to make children sterile, undermining the polio vaccination campaign and breaking trust.

In Ethiopia, rumours discouraged families from vaccinating their children because of fears of inducing sterility and disability,[506] highlighting suspicions of immunization side effects as a barrier to implementation. In Nigeria, fears stemming from an American conspiracy to induce HIV and infertility through the polio vaccine resulted in decreased acceptance in five northern states.[507] The potential harms of vaccines, such as the induction of sterility or disability and negative health effects on children, are widespread in LMICs.[508]

In Liberia, fears of vaccines because of past Ebola experiences deterred polio vaccine uptake. During Ebola outbreaks in the region, participants in Liberia "recounted how immunization teams had worn personal protective equipment and that this caused communities to be afraid" of polio immunization.[509(p.86)] Regardless of the widespread notion that vaccines prevent illnesses, having the term *vaccine* associated with Ebola triggered very real fears about vaccines, influencing people's perceptions of other vaccines.[509] The Ebola outbreak directly compromised the immunization efforts in Liberia. All planned national immunization campaigns (including polio) were halted for the outbreak's duration because of human resource constraints. Moreover, the fear of contracting the Ebola virus in health facilities may have prevented caregivers from pursuing immunization services for their children.[510] Misinformation, fear, and distrust in the efficacy of the vaccines could push individuals towards alternative traditional protections against poliovirus infections, rather than towards the polio vaccine.

How can fears or rumours be dealt with? The key is strategic communication around trust, such as the integral use or involvement of the community. Communities need to be active participants in an intervention rather than passive recipients of a campaign delivered by outsiders.

In a 2016 ethnographic study of seven countries,[511] researchers examined polio vaccine acceptance, refusal, and policy decisions supporting vaccination campaigns. A significant enabler for anticipating and dealing with fears and rumours was actively engaging town chiefs, elders, mothers, youth leaders, and local church leaders.

Influential opinions from interested parties, such as religious leaders and health professionals, can be closely tied to acceptance of the polio program, which can heavily influence parents' decision-making and hinder or strengthen program implementation.

The meaning and values attached to the intervention by health workers and opinion leaders in Uganda highlighted their influence since the public emulated their refusal to vaccinate their children.[512] Reservations about the intervention can be influenced by individuals who may be involved in the intervention or whose opinions may be perceived as credible.

Champions can facilitate intervention implementation. There have been records of health-focused champions endorsing the uptake of polio vaccination, thus positively influencing the decision-making process of participants across Angola, Ethiopia, Nigeria, and Rwanda.[511] Ground-level workers also cited the engagement of political and other leaders as reasons for increased acceptance of the polio vaccine.[511]

2. Inadequate Infrastructure Undermines Progress

The infrastructure surrounding campaigns is a necessary implementation component of polio programs. General infrastructural issues impede effective implementation and limit efforts to reach vulnerable populations.[513] Conversely, in the presence of good infrastructure and resource mobilization, the implementation of polio programs was deemed successful. Infrastructure was one of the seven themes that emerged from determinants of polio eradication in a global review.

One study from Nigeria highlighted that the general lack of basic necessities, including drug availability in hospitals and water service, was a barrier to future immunization uptake:[514] "Why will the government be chasing us with vaccine, when in the hospital the doctor ask us to pay for everything even headache drugs, why should I now let them give my children vaccine?"

In Niger, a team of researchers conducted community analyses to assess the social and cultural factors that affect the detection and reporting of disease cases in a surveillance system, using AFP. Eighty-seven percent of the nurses who were interviewed said that lack of access to healthcare for most people is a barrier to routine immunizations, and thus to AFP surveillance, leading to fewer opportunities for interfaces between healthcare staff and children who are at risk for polio. In addition, numerous respondents noted inaccessibility as impeding routine immunizations and AFP surveillance.[515]

In Ethiopia, shortage of vaccine and supplies, non-functionality of refrigerators, lack of training, cancellation of immunization sessions, and unavailability of health posts to deliver the services[516] are possible reasons for low immunization. Other reasons for low immunization coverage include shortages of cold chain equipment, inadequate number of trained health staff, and high staff turnover. Typically, one staff member conducts immunization in catchment populations.[516] In Nigeria, "lack of mobility is a major challenge. You definitely cannot carry out effective social mobilization work without mobility because you need to cut across many places. We do not have any vehicles attached to this department."[517]

The distance between caretakers and healthcare centres also has direct effects on immunization outcomes. Lack of access to immunization facilities in some hard-to-reach areas prove to be a barrier for childhood immunization. The inconvenience for caretakers to travel long distances to reach immunization centres increases incomplete vaccination series. Inadequate structure, arrangement, and coordination of immunization seasons at the health centre level are barriers as well.[516]

Strengthening the health financial system and building the technical capability of health workers are critical. Equipping health facilities with the necessary materials, including vaccines and supplies, and establishing more health centres and health posts with sufficient staff would be vital contributions to improving the situation. For example, in Uganda, there was increased accessibility to immunization because of nearby posts for National Immunization Days (NIDs). NIDs are "selected days when measles and polio vaccines as well as vitamin A supplements are given to children between the ages of 0–59 months and are extra doses which supplement and do not replace the doses received according to routine immunizations."[518] The NID posts facilitated individuals' participation in routine immunization campaigns because there were

"NID posts very near and within a short walking distance" from their homes.[512(p.367)]

Finally, community mapping of households supplemented with routine visits has aided in developing registries of pregnant women, creating registries of births, tracking newborn immunization status, and tracing defaulters to ensure they are appropriately immunized.[519]

The impact of a strong infrastructure is highlighted by a 2019 paper demonstrating how low coverage because of inadequate routine immunization systems results in poorer access to vaccination services and an inability to follow up with subsequent vaccine doses.[520] The lack of a strong framework surrounding routine immunization has the potential to influence polio vaccinations, because high levels of baseline routine immunization coverage strengthens vaccination efforts.[521] Growth in routine immunization coverage increases opportunities for interfaces between healthcare staff and children who are at risk for polio.[515]

3. Beliefs about the Intervention Must Be Recognized

Beliefs related to the intervention have been prominent in Africa's polio eradication initiatives. Negative beliefs about the polio vaccine emerged from cultural beliefs, religious conceptions, and inadequate awareness of the vaccine's purpose and effectiveness. However, increased knowledge and positive beliefs about the vaccine's efficacy facilitates vaccine acceptance and program implementation.

In Niger, the importance of cultural beliefs in the decision to reject the vaccine is highlighted through a discourse with nurses and opinion leaders, who report that many parents believe that paralysis is caused by a divine or spiritual intervention.[515]

The rituals of traditional healers, a well-respected aspect of Nigerian cultural practices, are seen to be the treatment for such diseases. Consequently, parents consult with a traditional healer before they visit healthcare centres, since they believe that simple drops of OPV cannot replace their powerful rituals.[522] The challenges to polio program uptake from a lack of information, ignorance, and illiteracy were highlighted in Nigeria.[514] For instance, in Nigeria, many refusal respondents mentioned "drinking of clean water as a way to avoid polio virus, [while] others identified [that] ways to protect against polio included proper care and belief in God."[515(p.3326)] The belief that vaccination was unnecessary was an indicator for refusal and thus was a barrier to intervention.[514]

In Nigeria, safety concerns and religious misconceptions regarding the vaccine included witchcraft accusations and the notion that Westernized medicines threaten religious credentials.[511] Abdullahi dan Fodio, a revered religious scholar, raised concerns over accepting medical aid from non-Muslim donors. This created religious tension as hospitals were viewed as having a Western agenda and attracted suspicion.[522] Another difficult perception to combat was the religious belief that health and illnesses are given from Allah (God) and "to complain of ill-health is to lodge a complaint against Him – which is almost unthinkable."[522(p.1141)] Although the Quran clearly states that Muslims have a religious obligation to preserve life, the perspective of the locals regarding immunization was confused because "how does immunizing a child help if health is preordained?"[522(p.1141)]

Conversely, there are issues with belief in the vaccine's ability to protect against polio, as was seen in Uganda, where people believed that "the major aim [of the vaccine] was to 'weaken' the disease and/or 'strengthen' the children's capability in fighting diseases."[512(p.367)] The misconception about the vaccine's ability to protect against polio also includes the notion that vaccines "strengthen the ability of children to fight most if not all childhood diseases," even though participants were unable to link specific vaccinations to protection/prevention against specific diseases.[512] An additional misconception is that polio vaccine protects against the other six immunizable diseases, along with pneumonia, malaria, and diarrhea, and people think that "attending for polio" is synonymous with attending for all immunization.[512]

Effective community engagement and the public's awareness of polio vaccines and the intervention, in general, were mentioned by two studies as a positive influence on the vaccine uptake.[509,511] According to a mother in Monrovia, "We don't worry about the measles and polio vaccine because we know it from before, from when the children were younger." A female leader from a focus group stated, "Mothers know about measles, they have been experiencing it, so for the vaccine they were happy to carry their children. They know its importance." Affirming the importance of vaccination, a mother in Nimba confirmed, "We can't deny the vaccine, we have seen measles kill children. If you see it with your own eyes, you believe."[509] Spreading of fake news and lack of information are among the main factors that contribute to low immunization coverage.[523]

Interviews with women in waiting rooms by Ndiaye and colleagues in health centres confirmed the importance of cultural beliefs: "The period from when parents start seeing a local healer to when they realize that there is no improvement and therefore decide to go to the health centre is 2–4 weeks, and hence the detection, reporting and investigation of AFP cases are either prevented or delayed."[515(p.93)]

4. Intervention Design Can Influence Acceptance and Coverage

Intervention design is most associated with the CFIR construct of design quality and packaging, defined as excellence in how the intervention is bundled, presented, and assembled. It speaks not only to the intervention but also to how it is presented.[248]

Intervention design is central to the polio vaccination program and matters not just for the vaccine itself but all the vaccination and programmatic efforts surrounding the vaccine, including the strategies to reach target populations. It involves all activities related to service delivery of the vaccinations, individuals administering the vaccines, and whether trusted and related communication programs align with the vaccination campaign.

If a vaccination program is communicated as essential and mandatory, it can increase vaccine uptake. For example, in Nigeria, it was noted that "a majority of the acceptors presented their children for vaccination because they had been told to do so" by health workers.[514(p.3325)] Healthcare professionals and vaccine providers play a role across various vaccine decision groups as they are trusted and influential sources. Their recommendations may influence hesitant parents to immunize their children.[524]

The impact of mandating vaccination, rather than making it optional, on uptake is further exemplified in the implementation of the polio vaccine. The guidelines deemed it to be mandatory rather than optional, which facilitated uptake. In 2017, Italy started enforcing mandatory childhood vaccinations, and the outcome of this law has been positive, with a 1% increase in polio vaccine uptake since. This also resulted in one-third of the previously unvaccinated children born between 2011 and 2015 being immunized. Currently, the poliovirus vaccine is mandatory in 10 countries (Belgium, Bulgaria, Croatia, Czech Republic, France, Hungary, Italy, Latvia, Poland, and Slovakia) and recommended in all others.[523]

A presumptive approach to vaccination is recommended by the CDC. Parents are significantly more likely to resist vaccine recommendations if the providers use a participatory approach such as "what do you want to do about the shots?" over a presumptive format "your child needs three vaccines today." Although presumptive initiation format may be associated with lower-rated visitation, it is still linked with higher parental vaccine acceptance at the end of the visit.[525]

A study found that vaccine-refusing households have fewer outgoing ties to vaccine-accepting households, indicating the clustering of vaccine-refusing households in spatially localized pockets. Since neighbourhood perceptions and recommendations play a role in acceptance or refusal, targeting vaccine-refusing social clusters through tailored communication strategies can improve vaccine acceptance of immunization programs for polio.[526]

Polio eradication relies on campaigns in which health workers administer vaccines to children under five, usually door to door. The frequency of the campaigns can affect outcomes. Having several polio campaigns could be a facilitator of implementation; one study revealed that many respondents asserted the effectiveness of several campaigns. For example, polio was eliminated from India in 2011 through a program of intense campaign activity – more than 10 per year in much of Bihar and Uttar Pradesh. There have been similar campaigns in Angola and Nigeria.[511]

Conclusion

Africa has made significant progress in the fight against polio, reaching a monumental milestone in 2020 with the eradication of wild polio. However, Africa continues its battle against other forms of polio. With the emergence of eight cases of wild poliovirus in 2022, the need to work diligently to ensure timely detection and quick outbreak response are more critical than ever. Several barriers still exist around polio immunization and its ultimate eradication. For the eradication efforts to be fruitful, these barriers, whether they exist on a personal or state/government level, must be acknowledged and addressed. Addressing personal barriers involves anticipating and recognizing fears and rumours and various beliefs about the vaccine. Obstacles at the state level revolve around infrastructure and how the vaccine is designed, packaged, and implemented vis-à-vis vaccination campaigns.

10
The Meningitis Vaccine Project: Remaking an Implementation Climate

The Global Roadmap to Defeat Meningitis demonstrates what can be accomplished when a global need is met with global action.

– Nikolaj Gilbert, president and CEO of PATH

In 1996 and 1997, sub-Saharan Africa experienced its historically largest meningitis epidemic. In 2000, global health leaders deemed a low-cost conjugate vaccine against group A *Neisseria meningitidis* possible. The next year, the Bill and Melinda Gates Foundation awarded a 10-year grant to establish the Meningitis Vaccine Project (MVP). The MVP team produced the vaccine MenAfriVac under the sustainable price of USD 0.50 per dose and in 2005 launched human clinical trials. Phase 1 enrolled 74 healthy adults in India, and in 2006, in response to a pandemic, phase 2 launched in Africa for a younger group. The next year, the vaccine was deemed safe and 20 times as potent as the previously marketed vaccine.

This chapter aims to evaluate the transformative impact of the MenAfriVac vaccine on the reduction of meningitis A epidemics in sub-Saharan Africa. It will explore key strategies and factors that contributed to the MVP and assess lessons gleaned from the MVP to understand their broader implications for the scale-up of health innovations in Africa.

By 2009, the MVP team was ready to request Indian licensure and WHO prequalification for use in Africa. MVP then built countries' capacity to integrate MenAfriVac into their health programs, and the WHO led the strengthening of disease surveillance and laboratory capacity for the most affected countries. E-learning tools were also designed for immunization managers in developing countries. The efforts were supported by the Yaoundé Declaration of 2008, as ministers of health of

Meningitis Belt countries committed to quickly introducing the vaccine and strengthening disease surveillance, control plans, and cross-border information sharing. In 2010, the vaccine received WHO prequalification, and at the end of the year, countrywide vaccination campaigns reached 20 million people. In 2011, the vaccine was launched in three additional countries, and by the end of 2016, it reached over 270 million people, ages 1 to 29, in 19 countries across sub-Saharan Africa. The vaccine quickly reduced meningitis A transmission and created herd immunity, with one dose providing immunity for as long as 10 years.

Meningococcal meningitis is a serious global health issue because of its high fatality rate if left untreated (up to 50%).[527] However, Africa historically has had the highest incidence of this infection, especially countries within the Meningitis Belt, which account for 84.6% of all cases within Africa.[528] This belt stretches from Senegal to Ethiopia and Somalia and includes 26 countries.[529]

In 2016, 2.8 million cases of meningitis occurred (all causes, not just bacterial) globally and 318,400 deaths. The African Meningitis Belt was the region with the highest mortality and incidence rates, with 6 of the 10 countries in the Belt.

Meningococcal meningitis is still very much an issue in Africa, especially since it seems to thrive in dry climates, commonly found in sub-Saharan Africa.[530] However, because of strong vaccination programs within developed countries, as well as the introduction of MenAfriVac, which targets the deadliest form of meningococcal meningitis in the Meningitis Belt, the prevalence and fatality rate of meningococcal meningitis has dropped globally.[530]

Countries within the Meningitis Belt commonly experienced endemics and epidemics in the past, which caused cases of meningococcal meningitis to fluctuate yearly. For example, 17 epidemics were reported from 2011 to 2017 in Africa, with many within the Belt; however, these epidemics were not caused by the common meningitis serotype A but by serotypes C (11 epidemics) and W (6 epidemics).[531] The countries affected were Niger, Nigeria, Burkina Faso, Ghana, Ethiopia, Togo, Benin, and Cameroon.[531] While these epidemics were relatively small individually, they led to a total of 30,000 cases; regardless, any epidemic can quickly get out of control if left untreated.[531]

For example, the largest recorded epidemic occurred in 1996–97 within the Belt, leading to over 250,000 cases and 50,000 deaths.[532] At the time, there was no MenAfriVac vaccine to prevent the epidemic. While there was a response by major organizations, including the WHO and the UN, few measures had been put in place to have prevented it. Certain reactive responses were put in too quickly, leading

Figure 10.1. Meningitis Milestones and Medical Breakthroughs over the Decades

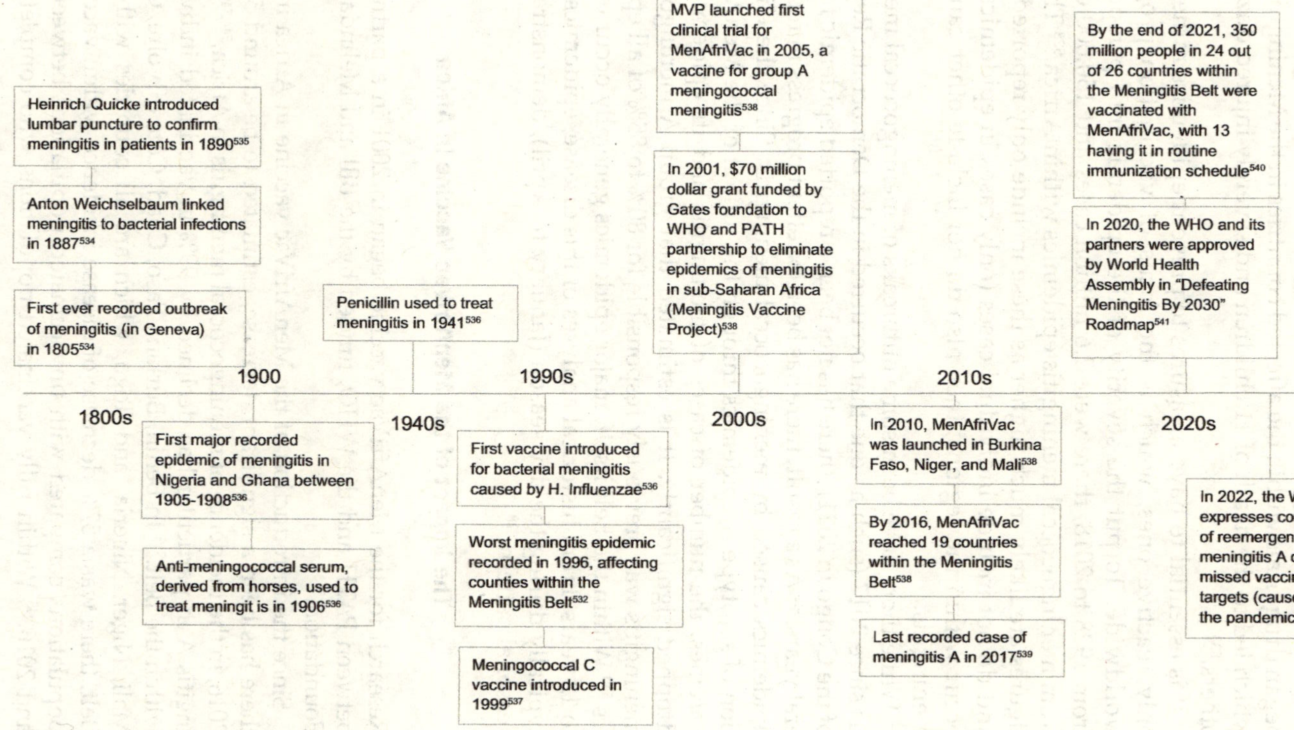
Heinrich Quicke introduced lumbar puncture to confirm meningitis in patients in 1890[535]
Anton Weichselbaum linked meningitis to bacterial infections in 1887[534]
First ever recorded outbreak of meningitis (in Geneva) in 1805[534]
1800s
1900
First major recorded epidemic of meningitis in Nigeria and Ghana between 1905-1908[536]
Anti-meningococcal serum, derived from horses, used to treat meningit is in 1906[536]
1940s
Penicillin used to treat meningitis in 1941[536]
1990s
First vaccine introduced for bacterial meningitis caused by H. Influenzae[536]
Worst meningitis epidemic recorded in 1996, affecting counties within the Meningitis Belt[532]
Meningococcal C vaccine introduced in 1999[537]
2000s
MVP launched first clinical trial for MenAfriVac in 2005, a vaccine for group A meningococcal meningitis[538]
In 2001, $70 million dollar grant funded by Gates foundation to WHO and PATH partnership to eliminate epidemics of meningitis in sub-Saharan Africa (Meningitis Vaccine Project)[538]
2010s
In 2010, MenAfriVac was launched in Burkina Faso, Niger, and Mali[538]
By 2016, MenAfriVac reached 19 countries within the Meningitis Belt[538]
Last recorded case of meningitis A in 2017[539]
2020s
By the end of 2021, 350 million people in 24 out of 26 countries within the Meningitis Belt were vaccinated with MenAfriVac, with 13 having it in routine immunization schedule[540]
In 2020, the WHO and its partners were approved by World Health Assembly in "Defeating Meningitis By 2030" Roadmap[541]
In 2022, the WHO expresses concerns of reemergence of meningitis A due to missed vaccination targets (caused by the pandemic)[542]

to further death. For example, Pfizer had introduced an antibiotic drug that was thought to treat meningitis in the 1996 epidemic and began drug trials within the affected countries in the Meningitis Belt, which led to the death of 11 children and severely injured dozens of others.[533]

It is essential to have measures to prevent epidemics rather than only reactive ones, which is the focus of vaccination programs worldwide. To put the severity of the epidemic into perspective, from 1928 to 2018, there were 2.6 million cases and 150,000 deaths from meningococcal meningitis epidemics within Africa.[528] The real figures are likely much higher as these include only reported cases and do not include individual cases (only cases in epidemics) that occur within the regions; they also do not include other causes of meningitis.

While there have been some outbreaks of meningococcal meningitis since 2017 (such as one that occurred in the Democratic Republic of the Congo in 2021), there has not been a reported epidemic for several years.[541] As a result, there has been excellent progress in reducing epidemics caused by meningococcal meningitis. Since the elimination of serotype A epidemics through the rollout of the MenAfriVac vaccines, the number of cases of meningitis and its epidemics has dropped significantly. It is estimated that group A meningococcal meningitis was previously responsible for 80% to 85% of all epidemics.[540] Within the Belt itself, major epidemics generally occur every 5 to 12 years. From historical analyses of this disease, epidemics occur typically during the dry season (January to April), demonstrating a seasonal pattern.[528]

The Impact of the MenAfriVac Vaccine in Africa

Research for the MenAfriVac vaccine began in 2001 in a partnership between PATH and the WHO, funded by the Bill and Melinda Gates Foundation.[543]

Since the introduction of the MenAfriVac vaccine in Africa in 2010, there has been a significant decrease, estimated to be around 57% by 2016, in the incidence of meningococcal meningitis in Africa.[544,545] Meningitis A in particular has declined by 99% in vaccinated individuals within the Belt.[545] In Benin, Burkina Faso, Chad, Côte d'Ivoire, Ghana, Mali, Niger, Nigeria, and Togo, which are all countries within the Belt, there was a 57% decrease of disease incidence within vaccinated populations compared with unvaccinated populations between 2010 and 2016.[545] Within fully vaccinated populations who completed the

MenAfriVac campaign in sub-Saharan Africa, there was a 99% decrease in the incidence of the meningococcal group A strain, which is responsible for most of the epidemics.[545] An estimated 350 million Africans in 24 out of 26 of the most high-risk countries (countries within the Meningitis Belt) have been vaccinated, which caused the cases of meningitis A to drop to only 80 globally in 2015.[539,543] All 26 countries in the Belt, since 2016, have provided the MenAfriVac vaccine, which has essentially led to eradicating meningitis A; since 2017, there have been no reported meningitis A cases.[539]

While MenAfriVac has decreased epidemics and outbreaks of meningitis by a significant margin, it's important to keep in mind that it does not protect against other serotypes of meningococcal meningitis. MenAfriVac is a monovalent vaccine that specifically protects against group A meningococcal meningitis; however, there are other types of meningococcal meningitis that it does not protect against. Even though the bacteria are the same species, they have different surface antigens.[546] Because of a shift in the prevalence of non-serotype A strains caused by herd immunity against the group A strain, meningococcal meningitis still remains a major burden for sub-Saharan Africa.[531]

This prevalence became apparent from 2011 to 2017, as all 17 epidemics during this time were due to non-serotype A strains.[531] Individual cases of meningococcal meningitis on other continents like Europe and the Americas are more commonly also caused by other serotypes, like B, C, and W; considering countries within these continents are generally more developed, this trend is positive for the countries within the Meningitis Belt.[544] Although serotype A was once responsible for 80% to 85% of all meningococcal epidemic cases, other serotypes still account for 15% to 20% of all cases, and there is currently no protection for them in the Meningitis Belt.[544]

Unfortunately, because of COVID-19, an estimated 50 million children missed their MenAfriVac vaccine; these 50 million children were targeted in vaccination campaigns, but the campaigns were delayed because of the COVID-19 pandemic. As a result, there has been a concern about the resurgence of meningitis A, the strain responsible for most previous outbreaks.[542]

It's important to continue vaccination campaigns to prevent future outbreaks, especially because of the severity of meningitis. Currently, research is being done on an affordable pentavalent vaccine that will protect against other serotypes of meningococcal meningitis, which are responsible for 15% to 20% of other meningococcal cases. This will decrease the incidence even further.[543,544]

Lessons from the MVP

Lesson 1: How Tension for Change and Commitment of African Leaders Led to a Positive Start for the MVP

In the years before the MVP kicked off, there was a strong tension for change – the degree to which involved parties perceived the current situation as intolerable or requiring change. The evident tension was translated into the commitment and advocacy of African leaders to bring attention and urgency to addressing the burden of meningitis A.

Tension for change is a critical construct of the Consolidated Framework of Implementation Research, where there is dissatisfaction with the status quo, which in this case were the repeated outbreaks and deaths from meningitis. The construct *tension for change* is part of the inner setting domain of the framework that relates to the characteristics of the implementing organization and its partners, which can influence implementation. To delineate the barriers and facilitators to the MPV, a qualitative study was conducted with 18 key individuals involved with the project.[547] One person from the WHO Africa involved in the project deployment captured the evidence for this strong tension for change:

> I think the first facilitator or enabling factor was the decision by the then head of state of Burkina Faso, then President Compaoré, to make a call, a specific call for a vaccine to be developed against meningitis – which was really a plague, because it was simply causing a lot of illness and of course a lot of deaths in sub-Saharan Africa, across the Meningitis Belt. So this call by the president of the region, which was also supported by other leaders of Mali, Chad, Niger, and other African leaders from West Africa, I think was a major factor because for the first time we had a call by a group of countries for a vaccine to be developed specifically to address a disease in the region. So that's one enabling factor.

It is difficult to create tension for change when none exists, but in the case of the MVP, the tension for change was not without reason. The disease outbreaks were devastating, thus pressuring African leaders to find a solution. According to an interviewee from the World Health Organization Regional Office for Africa, "Meningitis has caused a lot of death, a lot of outbreaks. It was like, you know, every year having a major outbreak in one of the active countries or several active countries within the Meningitis Belt. It was well known within the region, so it was quite a big concern for government." Therefore, once the vaccine was made available, the majority of governments within the Belt were interested in introducing the vaccine.

From 1928 to 2018, the highest case numbers were reported in 1996, and within this same period, Burkina Faso suffered the highest number of deaths in the Meningitis Belt.[528]

During this time, there were other infections and health problems in Burkina Faso and across the Meningitis Belt. However, the other infections were not seen as a top priority by the countries, and the risk of epidemics, which were fresh in the memory of many countries through the massive 1996 outbreak, was an important trigger.

One of the reasons for the success was that the demand came from African leaders. In other words, the initiative originated from the African ministers of health who expressed a clear need for the vaccine, rather than it being imposed from outside sources. This local demand played a crucial role in driving the project's effectiveness.

Through a partnership of the leaders of the African countries, they made a verbal commitment to see the project forward because of the magnitude and threat this had for their nations and their peoples, with the cases and deaths five years earlier still present in their minds.

The critical need identified by African leaders for a meningitis serotype A vaccine stemmed from the consequences of disease outbreaks that were going through sub-Saharan Africa periodically. In other words, the African heads of state somewhat demanded that the WHO find a solution.

In addition, the tension for change expanded through advocacy from Burkina Faso to other countries in the Meningitis Belt. In the words of an individual involved in the deployment and governance of the project:

> Yeah, making advocacy to the other country that has leading all these African and WHO liaised with the president of Faso to be a kind of godfather for these future projects in the benefit of the population. I think the community engagement in my sense was very important, and we had a chance to liaise with this authority and say, okay, look at the president of Burkina Faso agreed to be kind of, kind of what can I say kind of godfather, you know, that kind of sponsoring all the African.

However, advocacy and commitment need to be sustained to ensure that countries are aware of the need to introduce the vaccine into their routine program to reduce or eliminate epidemics and ensure long-term protection in the community.

Lesson 2: Strong Transformational Leadership Translated into a Successful MVP Campaign

Formally appointed internal implementation leaders were critical in successful vaccine implementation. The project director of the MVP provided excellent leadership and expertise.

According to a partner actively involved in the project,

> I give great credit to Marc Laforce and his efforts and his ability to bring groups together to address this issue. He had a real challenge, because most of the major manufacturers of conjugate vaccines weren't really interested in this particular project, so he had to find an alternative solution, a public-private partnership. And, once he was chosen as the leader to move the initiative forward, there were huge challenges, but he was able to overcome those challenges in a very creative way.

In addition to Laforce's effective leadership, he brought the right team together, translating it into a need to take care of all involved parties. He pushed to develop the vaccine and ensured that that development aligned with the country's needs and was affordable and cost-effective for the recipient countries.

A strong director is a crucial driver of a large-scale project, especially one with a common goal for all the partnerships. It helped that there was a charismatic leader. Colleagues describe Laforce as having a "strong focus" and "relentless drive," which were very helpful to the project.

One critical element of Dr. Laforce's leadership was his vision and goal orientation. According to a colleague who worked with him, "He has set himself a ten-year goal. 'I am going to make sure that meningitis is no longer a problem in Africa.' So that is what I can say about that."

Finally, the director was a great facilitator because he trusted the competence of the staff and partners and understood delegation. He was very good at picking people whose expertise would be helpful and contribute positively. There was a global population of experts that he drew upon, and he was able to do that effectively.

A characteristic of effective leadership is responsible delegation and leveraging technical expertise through recruitment. The technical expertise sought and provided throughout the implementation stages was a critical facilitator to successfully implementing the vaccine program, which was achieved through the engagement of product experts, the Expanded Programme on Immunisation department of the WHO, and epidemiologists.

Lesson 3: External Change Agents Were Vital to Sustaining Momentum and Overcoming Hurdles

The involvement of multiple partners and interested groups – such as donors, agencies, government, and communities – was highlighted as a critical facilitator to the success of the MVP. How well these key partners worked together was primarily the result of strong leadership as described in the previous lesson.

These agents formally influenced and facilitated the intervention decisions in a desirable direction. There was GAVI, UNICEF, the CDC, Doctors Without Borders/Médecins Sans Frontières, and the CDC Foundation. There were also African governments, which not only made a commitment but involved their ministries of health.

According to one of the project implementers, choosing the right people at the beginning was critical:

> We were challenged on that a number of times, set up an expert panel, and did quite a rigorous selection process that I think helped us end up with the right partners. The expert groups and the governance groups, the vaccine introduction groups that we set up from the very beginning making sure that we had the right people involved in, in the key decisions of the project, I think really facilitated its success.

There was a strong partnership with a defined role for each of those partners and quite an amicable coordinated approach to it: "There's different touchpoints, we're in constant communication, also, because GAVI is very much an alliance so it's part of the nature of GAVI as an organization to work very closely with partners as well." There was the private sector, the Serum Institute in India, and the public sector, which were the governments of African countries together with WHO Africa.

The value of the WHO cannot be overemphasized in terms of providing access to the country's ministries of health; they are on-the-ground surveillance. The WHO's respected reputation was critical. Although a few people might have concerns about the WHO and the bureaucracy, there were advantages to working with an organization that had links throughout the world and was highly respected, particularly the African Regional Offices and Country Offices. The WHO was also instrumental in facilitating regulatory approvals and approving new vaccines, and it had links with nationals in each of the countries to introduce and roll out the vaccine. The WHO's role was a factor in making this successful by bringing together the partners.

There was also PATH, which was instrumental in product development expertise, commercialization agreements, legal aspects, and robust management infrastructure, which was an excellent complement to the WHO.

Although the MVP had a large number of partners, there was still a great deal of unified vision. It was an opportunity for partners and governments to collaborate and work together with that same voice and vision, which contributed greatly to the project's success. According to someone in the project involved in exploratory/pre-clinical, distribution/delivery of the vaccine, "So, getting the right people together was really the key. The variety of partners/stakeholders was critical."

Several partners came in at different times. Some of these partners, such as Serum Institute of India, had a role to play throughout the project. Some others had a role at a particular time and then no role later, but the project continued to keep them involved, generating a sense of partnership.

Funding flexibility and autonomy early in the project were necessary. According to the project personnel, "The Gates Foundation did not have adequate human capacity and decided to fund the project in one go. Therefore, from the outset, the money was available. There was no chance for the donor to micromanage or try to influence the process. The money was out." In other words, the project received a significant amount of relatively flexible funding. This allowed the project's leaders and partners to be creative in moving forward, which was an essential driver for success.

Lesson 4: Key Attributes That Made It Easier to Procure and Distribute Vaccines Were Critical

Key attributes of the vaccine were critical for successful implementation, including the cost, single dose, and stability of the freeze-dried vaccine.

First, the manufacturer (Serum Institute of India) was willing to develop a cost-effective vaccine and was the perfect partner. The program worked to provide a vaccine that met the specific need of African countries: it was inexpensive compared with other vaccines. It was important to respect financial constraints; these were developing countries in which the epidemics were most common.

Second, the needs were clearly identified, including the medical needs. They needed a fully efficient vaccine against meningitis serotype A in one single dose that was easy to administer.

Finally, it was a vaccine that could be provided outside the cold chain, which was critical to getting it out to people in remote areas, and it was affordable for African countries. These issues were discussed upfront in the development of the project among partners. Vaccine deployment can be challenging in areas of Africa without electricity. If a vaccine is in the refrigerator and in the morning is taken out, there are only four hours in which it can be used to vaccinate without having ice.

However, it is crucial to recognize the challenges encountered in vaccine development. There were complexities, delays, and setbacks related to the science of developing a new vaccine, a conjugate vaccine. A conjugate vaccine is complex; during its development, unexpected things can happen that must be resolved.

The usual way to create a vaccine is to have Big Pharma make it, and it was apparent early on that this route would not be available. A major hurdle that needed to be overcome for this project was the lack of interest by Big Pharma in partnering for the meningitis serotype A vaccine. Manufacturers of conjugate vaccines were not interested in such a project; therefore, a public-private partnership model was necessary.

The strategy was to adapt that platform into a new type of vaccine to prevent serogroup meningitis, and that was a conjugation technology. Some patents were held by the companies, but they were not really interested in participating, so the technology was actually made available from the US Food and Drug Administration (FDA) to the Serum Institute of India.

A group working extensively with the FDA had developed a technology for conjugation of the protein with a polysaccharide, which is the foundation for the vaccine. That technology was made available to Marc LaForce and his partners, put together for the creation of this vaccine, at no cost. That was fundamentally a critical issue, how to get the intellectual property needed to create the vaccine that was ultimately manufactured and used.

According to a person involved in the exploratory/pre-clinical and a consultant for the project: "The adaptability through the FDA-approved technology transfer to the Serum Institute of India. These, among others, were crucial facilitators of the successful development, production, and implementation of the vaccine program. Using their network of people that they'd built up, you know. The FDA link was crucial for the conjugation technology."

Conclusion

Before the MenAfriVac vaccine, there were not many preventative measures for meningitis A in Africa, and quickly implemented reactive responses created more fatalities and injuries. Since the vaccine's introduction in 2010, meningococcal meningitis decreased by 99% among vaccinated individuals, with no reported cases in 2017. There are four key lessons from the MVP to guide and facilitate the implementation of similar endeavours and to overcome barriers. First, strong tension for change and the commitment of African leaders to advance the project positively launched the MVP. Thus, advocacy and commitment were crucial in ensuring the vaccine was integrated into routine healthcare. Second, transformational leadership was responsible for the success of the MVP campaign. The MVP director, Marc LaForce, provided excellent leadership and expertise, recruited the right team, trusted the competence of his staff, delegated, and drew on their technical and other expertise. A third important lesson is that external change agents were vital to sustaining momentum and overcoming hurdles. The carefully selected partners and involved parties worked together under solid leadership with clearly defined roles to influence and facilitate intervention decisions in a favourable direction. Despite the length and period of their involvement, project partners were kept engaged, and the team enjoyed funding flexibility and autonomy. Finally, critical attributes of the vaccine, like its cost, single dose, and stability, made it successful, as it became easier to procure, distribute, and administer.

11
Human Papillomavirus Campaign: A Success Story in Rwanda

The first human papillomavirus (HPV) vaccine was commercially available in 2006 and was produced by Merck & Co.[548] This vaccine was found to protect against strains that caused 70% of cervical cancers and 90% of anogenital warts worldwide.[548]

However, one of the most considerable barriers to moving from the vaccine production stage to the implementation in LMICs is the cost, which can initially be USD 400 for a three-series dose.[548] Because of this significant barrier, organizations such as GAVI negotiated a decreased cost per dose of USD 4.50 to support African countries in 2013.[548]

The first nationwide rollout of the HPV vaccine in sub-Saharan Africa began in 2011, despite being widely available since 2006.[549] While some countries had more success than others, progress in national immunization programs was delayed for financial and technical resources reasons, with a significant hit during the COVID-19 pandemic, when vaccine supply shortages arose.[549]

In 2016, the vaccine alliance and non-profit organization GAVI approved an accelerated HPV vaccine program in which it would scale up vaccination within its first year in cohorts of girls ages 9 to 14 years in 27 countries, such as Rwanda.[550,551]

This chapter aims to assess the effectiveness and challenges of HPV vaccine rollout in Africa, with a particular emphasis on Rwanda's implementation strategy and its implications.

The Burden of Mortality/Morbidity of HPV Infection and Cervical Cancer in Africa

While the worldwide prevalence of HPV infection is estimated to be 11% to 12%, sub-Saharan Africa has disproportionally higher rates of 24%.[552] Poverty is known to be a significant barrier, both directly in accessing healthcare (e.g., pap smear screening) and indirectly as a measure of overall poor health.[553] In 2018, over 85% of deaths from HPV-related cancers were in LMICs, where it is estimated it will rise to 90% in 2030.[553] In particular, adolescent girls (who account for 19% of the population in South Africa) are at significantly high risk for HPV infection because of statistically poor sexual and reproductive outcomes at this age.[549]

Based on 2020 estimates, 415.49 million women ages 15 years and older are at risk of developing cervical cancer in Africa.[554] The annual number of new cervical cancer cases in Africa is 117,316, with an annual mortality of 76,745 from the disease.[554] Cervical cancer is the second-most-frequent cancer among women in Africa.[554]

In 2020, the highest regional incidence and mortality rates of cervical cancer were in sub-Saharan Africa. Elevated rates occur more specifically in Eastern Africa, Southern Africa, and Middle Africa.[555] Eastern Africa held the highest age standardized incidence rate of cervical cancer worldwide, with 40.1 per 100,000 women, with Southern Africa not far behind at 36.4 per 100,000 women.[555] Of these regions, Eastern Africa had an age standardized mortality rate of 28.6 per 100,000 women. Southern Africa reported a rate of about 20.6 per 100,000 women.[555]

Eastern Africa experiences the highest burden with 54,560 annual cases of cervical cancer. Northern Africa has the lowest among African regions at 6971 annual cases.[554] A large portion of cases within Eastern Africa are in Tanzania, making up 10,241 annual cases.[554] Southern Africa experiences a burden of 12,333 cases; however, 10,702 of the cervical cancer cases are in South Africa.[554] Furthermore, Nigeria makes up almost half of Western Africa's burden of disease, having 12,075 annual cases.[554] Mortality rates are more than half of all annual cases for both Nigeria and Tanzania.

A study in Northern Africa from 1993 to 2006 showed a decreasing trend in cervical cancer in Tunisia.[556] The declines have been a result of national screening programs, changes in sexual behaviour, and use of barrier contraception.[556] A similar trend was observed in Algeria for 1986 to 2010, which has also been attributed to screening programs.[557] Conversely, using 10 population-based cancer registries from eight countries in sub-Saharan Africa, a study by Jedy-Agba and colleagues[558] examined trends in the incidence of cervical cancer over 10 to 25 years. Results of the study found a high and increasing burden of cervical cancer in Eastern Africa over the examined time period.[558] The only country exhibiting declining trends from this study was Mauritius.[558] In 2010–14, a population-wide cytology screening program was introduced, which the declines may be attributable to.[558]

Figure 11.1. Key Milestones in HPV Vaccine Availability and Implementation in Africa, 2006–22

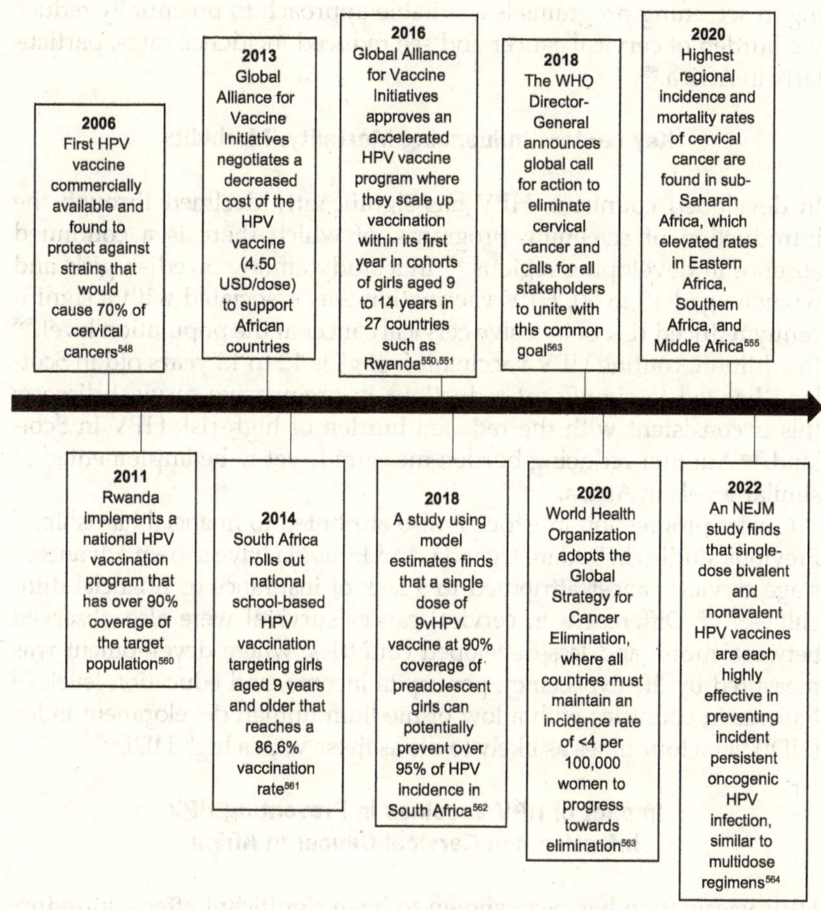

2006
First HPV vaccine commercially available and found to protect against strains that would cause 70% of cervical cancers[548]
2013
Global Alliance for Vaccine Initiatives negotiates a decreased cost of the HPV vaccine (4.50 USD/dose) to support African countries
2016
Global Alliance for Vaccine Initiatives approves an accelerated HPV vaccine program where they scale up vaccination within its first year in cohorts of girls aged 9 to 14 years in 27 countries such as Rwanda[550,551]
2018
The WHO Director-General announces global call for action to eliminate cervical cancer and calls for all stakeholders to unite with this common goal[563]
2020
Highest regional incidence and mortality rates of cervical cancer are found in sub-Saharan Africa, which elevated rates in Eastern Africa, Southern Africa, and Middle Africa[555]
2011
Rwanda implements a national HPV vaccination program that has over 90% coverage of the target population[560]
2014
South Africa rolls out national school-based HPV vaccination targeting girls aged 9 years and older that reaches a 86.6% vaccination rate[561]
2018
A study using model estimates finds that a single dose of 9vHPV vaccine at 90% coverage of preadolescent girls can potentially prevent over 95% of HPV incidence in South Africa[562]
2020
World Health Organization adopts the Global Strategy for Cancer Elimination, where all countries must maintain an incidence rate of <4 per 100,000 women to progress towards elimination[563]
2022
An NEJM study finds that single-dose bivalent and nonavalent HPV vaccines are each highly effective in preventing incident persistent oncogenic HPV infection, similar to multidose regimens[564]

Vaccination against HPV is known to be the most effective preventative measure for cervical cancer.[558] HPV vaccines have been widely accessible in more developed regions since 2006; however, the nationwide rollout of HPV vaccination in sub-Saharan Africa did not occur until 2011.[558] As a result, the observed impact on population-level incidence rates may not be detectable in the next few decades, until generations of girls vaccinated reach maximum risk age.[558,559] Thus, the combined integration of HPV vaccine programs with HPV-based testing in screening programs is a suitable approach to potentially reduce the burden of cervical cancer and see reduced incidence rates, particularly in Africa.[559]

Key Factors Influencing Mortality/Morbidity

In developed countries, HPV has significantly declined through the introduction of screening programs, of which there is a continued absence in developing regions.[558] In a study among Swedish girls and women aged 10 to 30, HPV vaccination was associated with a significantly reduced risk of invasive cervical cancer at the population level.[565] In addition, routine HPV vaccination of girls 12 to 13 years old in Scotland has led to significant reductions in preinvasive cervical disease; this is consistent with the reduced burden of high-risk HPV in Scotland.[566] Another reducing burden measure is yet to be implemented at similar levels in Africa.

Cancer progression in Africa is also attributed to financial hardship.[567] Previous studies in Sudan, Uganda, and Ethiopia have shown advanced-stage cervical cancer attributed to a lack of insurance or financial difficulties.[567,568] Differences in cervical cancer survival were also observed between more- and less-developed countries, where development was measured by life expectancy, per capita income, and education levels.[569] Patients in countries with a low or medium human development index (HDI) were four times as likely to die as those with a high HDI.[569]

Impact of HPV Vaccines in Preventing HPV Infection and Cervical Cancer in Africa

HPV vaccination has been shown to have significant effects in reducing the incidence of HPV infection and cervical cancer.[562] A modelling analysis study in South African endemic regions showed the effects of HPV vaccination on HPV infection and cervical cancer. As noted, the study projected that a single-dose 9vHPV vaccination at 90% coverage of preadolescent girls could prevent over 95% of HPV incidence in South Africa.[562] A decrease in cervical cancer incidence and mortality followed these reductions in HPV prevalence. The study also found that lower coverage rates of 50% and 70% of preadolescent girls may significantly impact the cervical cancer burden.[562]

Another study performed a randomized, double-blinded, controlled trial of a nonavalent or bivalent HPV vaccination to study the efficacy of vaccination against HPV infection in Kenyan women ages 15 to 20 years. The study took place between December 2018 and June 2021. The study demonstrated a protection rate of 97.5% against HPV infection for two separate HPV vaccines.[564]

A study in Botswana displayed a high prevalence of HPV in women with and without HIV.[570] The HPV virus genotypes included strains that are targeted by a quadrivalent HPV vaccine. These findings push for the importance of HPV vaccination and will allow for evaluation of future studies in determining the impact of HPV vaccine on HPV infection and cervical cancer.

A mathematical analysis study estimated the impact that HPV vaccination can have on HPV infection and cervical cancer incidence in Africa, specifically Kenya. From the model estimation, HIV prevalence would reach 0.3% in 2070 as compared with the current 6.5% among women.[571] Cervical cancer incidence is also estimated to reduce by 70% to 85%, depending on the cohort age group being administered a nonvalent HPV vaccine.[571] These show the significant effects that HPV vaccination can have on reduction of cervical cancer incidence over the next half-century in Kenya.

Finally, a modelling and analysis study using demographic figures along with aging populations exhibit HPV vaccination's health benefits in decreasing the burden of cervical cancer.[572] More specifically, the study estimated that Africa would have the most significant benefit from HPV vaccination upscaling with 28 cases, 23 deaths, and 470 disability-adjusted life years averted per 1000 vaccinated girls.[572]

One of the first reported studies on the impact of HPV vaccine in preventing HPV infection and cervical cancer in Africa was conducted by Felix Sayinzoga and colleagues.[573] Their study utilized repeated cross-sectional surveys involving sexually active young women in Rwanda, comparing data collected before the vaccine's introduction (2013–14) with data from after its rollout (2019–20). The results indicated a notable adjusted vaccine effectiveness of 47% against the HPV types included in the vaccine (HPV6, 11, 16, and 18).[573,574] While the full effects of HPV vaccination on cervical cancer incidence and mortality in Africa will not be observable for several years, there is an urgent need to promote and strengthen HPV vaccination efforts across Africa.

Key Lessons from the HPV Campaign Implementation in Rwanda

Lesson 1: A Robust Partnership with Relevant External Organizations Garners Success and Overcomes Resource Hurdles

Partnerships with external organizations were critical to providing access to HPV vaccines and other resources and to supporting Rwanda's capacity building during its HPV campaign.

In the middle of Rwanda's long rainy season in 2011, and less than a year after President Paul Kagame's election for a second term, the Rwandan Government launched the HPV vaccination campaign together with companies Merck and QIAGEN. The campaign also included HPV testing as part of a comprehensive cancer prevention program, which led to more than 90% of eligible girls being vaccinated with three doses of Gardasil.[575]

Rwanda's close partnership and collaboration with Merck helped prevent many barriers from arising. Millions of doses were provided, which was critical to Rwanda kick-starting its immunization program smoothly and creating a public-private community partnership.

Collaboration with external organizations, including GAVI, the Pan American Health Organization, the WHO, UNICEF, and others, was a key facilitator in Rwanda's HPV campaign rollout and implementation. GAVI was instrumental in ensuring the long-term sustainability of the program. These external partnerships were helpful in areas including technical expertise and information sharing, funding opportunities, and vaccine accessibility.

A study was conducted on the HPV vaccine project in Rwanda. The study interviewed key players in its implementation.[576] A researcher in cervical cancer pathology, who supported the national government, commented on what led to the HPV campaign's success:

> I think the government of Rwanda made it its primary responsibility and has actually aimed to make sure they invest of course, in partnership with all the partners who are international – even local – in trying to improve the health of citizens – so that's the biggest factor in my opinion. ... Rwanda tries to tap into most of these initiatives that are internationally available, including people in Gavi, partnerships with WHO, and partnerships with everyone that fund anything that can actually improve the lives of citizens. So I think those are the things in my opinion that led to where we are now.

Lesson 2: Rwanda's Grade-Based Vaccine Selection Was a Critical Factor to Its Successful Campaign

Rwanda's grade-based vaccine campaign in schools enabled the country to reach its intended target population efficiently. Compared with the proposed age-based strategy by the WHO, this grade-based strategy worked far better in the Rwandan context and was a key facilitator in the success of the HPV campaign.

HPV vaccination guidelines generally define target by age, which is the international norm. However, according to several implementers of the HPV vaccination in Rwanda, it may be challenging to establish girls' ages in some contexts.

Therefore, the grade-based strategy resolved the issue of various ages existing in a specific grade, which can be a challenge in implementing the age-based strategy. In some situations, particularly in rural areas, the exact ages of girls cannot be known. A demonstration project in Uganda showed problems in identifying girls through an age-based program.[577,578] Therefore, it was less cumbersome to implement the HPV campaign with girls based on grade and achieve higher coverage.

Rwanda has exceptionally high enrolment rates in schools, which makes schools an ideal setting for HPV immunizations. For example, the enrolment for primary education in 2011, the year of the HPV campaign, was 94.3% for boys and 97.5% for girls.[579]

The grade-based strategy was straightforward for the implementers to start the program. They decided that the HPV vaccine would be delivered to girls mainly on school premises through two-day campaigns conducted three times a year. This was a key driver of the campaign and one of the significant decisions that the Ministry of Health made, as it enabled the government to access the most eligible girls at the time, particularly with such a high enrolment for girls.

In schools, adolescent girls were educated on HPV infection and cervical cancer, combined with nutritional education, family planning, peer education, and hygiene awareness. These activities assisted in obtaining consent for vaccination, spreading knowledge on cervical cancer, and decreasing the ongoing misconceptions and rumours. In other words, organizing this campaign through schools was less arduous.

According to a researcher and trainer in vaccinology, who focused on the vaccine introduction: "They [Ministry of Health] understood that best approach would be to deliver the vaccines through a school-based strategy and across as there is a general understanding that targeting the adolescent girls using an age-based strategy is not as effective as using the grade-based."

Lesson 3: Strong Political Will and Leadership Engagement Were Crucial in Getting the Project Off to the Right Start

The Rwandan government's political will and leadership engagement were crucial in influencing vaccine acceptance across the country.

Political will translates into seeking and securing external partnerships, continually engaging with national partners and advocates, promoting the synthesis of scientific evidence to support the impact of HPV vaccines, and diffusing effective communication strategies related to the campaign across various platforms.[580]

According to a person who led the HPV introduction in several African and Asian countries, including Rwanda: "So the biggest facilitator is political will. ... It is sold as a vaccine against cancer, and cancer of the cervix is one of the leading cancers. This is second to breast cancer in female mortality from cancers in Africa. And in most countries, it's the leading cause of cancer deaths. At least. All communities know somebody who has had cancer, so it was very easy to sell politically and also at community level."

In Rwanda, the implementation was linked to the Minister of Health, who acted as a champion in the process. This involvement ensured the implementation was successful and had a great deal of momentum, which was important in engendering strong political will and engaging communities.

Public trust in government health programs is high in Rwanda, enabling the HPV vaccine to be introduced with support. When something comes from the government, the population trusts it; this is another area that was a strong facilitator for the project. This is not surprising because in a CIVICUS Civil Society Index Analytical Country Report for Rwanda in 2011, the country and the government had a high level of public trust, with the leader of the country at 84.2% and the government at 63%.

However, when it comes to political parties, television, labour unions, the press, and companies, the trust level drops considerably to between 12% and 21%.

According to Mark Feinberg from Merck, "Rwanda is an incredible country in its commitment to national health. If it wasn't possible in Rwanda, we knew it wouldn't be possible anywhere else."[581]

Lesson 4: Intersectoral Collaboration Leveraged All of Rwanda's Assets for an Effective Campaign

Fostering intersectoral collaboration between formally appointed leaders, champions, and external change agents was vital in facilitating the success of the HPV campaign in Rwanda.

The collaboration and engagement between various national parastatals, including the ministries of Rwanda and the Ministry of Health, Education, and Gender and Family Promotion, allowed for the sharing of resource information. The collaborative work between the different ministries and government departments, as well as the health sector, acted as an enabler for this intervention. Establishing clear governance structures at all levels of immunization programs proved to be highly useful. Effective partnership and collaboration among government ministries – such as Education, Local Government, and Gender and Family Promotion – alongside the Ministry of Health, facilitated the successful mobilization of health programs. This collaborative approach made implementation more efficient and streamlined.[576]

In addition to partnerships between the ministries of health and the expanded immunization program, there was collaboration between the ministries of education and the ministries of social development, which informed on service delivery systems.

One significant characteristic of Rwanda's approach to health is that the social determinants of health are deliberately dealt with through multisectoral actions and are implemented by more than one sector. It has created national clusters, which are responsible for ensuring joint planning, monitoring, and evaluation interventions that are cross-cutting.[582]

In addition, intersectoral collaboration was extended to engaging women's groups, particularly by the First Lady, who played a significant role by going into the field, such as the district hospitals, and garnering support for the campaign. A key factor in Rwanda's successful vaccine implementation was strong political will, particularly from the First Lady, along with advocacy from women's rights groups and NGOs. These organizations framed the vaccine as a women's rights and equity issue, which contributed to its rapid national rollout and scale up. These champions of the HPV campaign created increased dialogue about the HPV vaccine. Moreover, change agents, such as community health workers, provided the human resources needed to reach the target population outside schools.[576]

The intersectoral collaboration is best captured by a statement made by a lead researcher who supported the monitoring and evaluation activities across health centres in Rwanda:

> When the HPV vaccination program was introduced in Rwanda so there was really a good support from so many stakeholders and I will start with leadership from high level. So, I remember I have got even the launch movie which was eventually attended by First Lady of the country. So this was something really very interesting to have a high-level person to come for the launching. And it shows not alone because actually shows together with the Minister of Health shows together with the former minister of Local Government, the former

> minister of education so you can understand when you have got this kind of personality in an event. So, it is very easy for people to follow the instruction they're giving, because everyone at that time was giving a good speech encouraging and motivating the population too to comply with the vaccination. Because we have good chance here in Rwanda. When something is coming from government. It is always trusted by the population, this is also another area in which I can say that it is an enabler, but also we cannot forget the health system we have here in Rwanda.

Together, the engagement of these individuals and groups contributed to the success of the HPV campaign in Rwanda.

Lesson 5: The Varied Nature of the HPV Vaccine Rollout Sensitization and Communication Was Vital in Its Implementation

The execution of the HPV vaccine rollout, including the sensitization and communication strategies, the catch-up campaign strategy, and the strategy to reach the out-of-school target population, were key factors influencing the success of the campaign.

Sensitization and communication strategies for the HPV vaccine rollout were crucial in addressing the misconceptions and fears felt by parents and caregivers, because knowledge and beliefs about the HPV vaccine were significant barriers to achieving effective implementation.[576] Before launching the HPV vaccine campaign, various communication channels were used to spread awareness, including TV, radio, social media, phones, and chatroom sessions. Social mobilization efforts involved influential figures like the First Lady, who appeared on TV and radio to emphasize the importance and impact of the HPV vaccine. Additionally, local authorities, leaders, and teachers were engaged to help convey the message and ensure wide community reach.

The multiple channels of communication were critical enablers and consolidated as one of the CFIR constructs: *networks and communications*. According to one of the key players in the monitoring and evaluation of the HPV vaccine in Rwanda at the onset of its launch, "so many radios, including the community radio. So, through mass media it is very easy. … community workers are now very well equipped with cell phones. So many kinds of information provided so there was always a mass media campaign, meetings, and the training of teachers and all stakeholders."

In addition, the implementers ensured a continual intensive social and community mobilization campaign that did not focus on one target, one particular person, or one end user but was varied.

A key communication message was framing the vaccine as an important tool to prevent sexually transmitted infections and cancer, which was key to increasing its acceptability among local people through community sensitization and mass media.

Other African Countries

As of 2023, 27 African countries had implemented the HPV vaccine into their national immunization schedules, targeting girls between the ages of 9 and 14. In November 2023, Togo became the newest country to join this effort, following Nigeria's introduction of the vaccine a month earlier.[583]

South Africa successfully rolled out a national school-based HPV vaccination program in 2014, which targeted grade 4 girls that were ages 9 years or older.[561] This program vaccinated over 350,000 girls in over 16,000 public schools, which proportionally translated to having 94.6% of schools reached with a 86.6% vaccination coverage of those eligible.[561] The campaign's success depended on careful planning, clear scheduling, a receptive target population, and effective coordination.[561] Interview data showed that a strong political commitment to results enormously helped the healthcare staff, coordinators, and other involved parties to deliver results.[561] Aside from its success, challenges to implementing the campaign included obtaining informed consent, storage capacity, onsite management, and the general spread of misinformation via social media.[561]

A pilot HPV vaccination program was conducted from 2013 to 2015 in eastern Kenya by the Ministry of Health, where 22,500 girls in class 4 and between the ages of 9 and 12 years received two doses of the HPV vaccine.[584] The uptake was considered successful at 96% and was used as an indicator to roll out the HPV vaccine by incorporating it into the routine immunization schedules of 10-year-old girls.[563] A main factor for the high uptake was the program being school based, as schools were considered better for vaccination programs to target SAC and adolescents.[584] Furthermore, parents and caregivers had higher acceptance of the vaccine because teachers are seen as trusted custodians who look after students' welfare.[584] Teachers' attitude and knowledge were a significant factor in ensuring the success of the vaccination program.[584]

In 2019, Kenya joined 115 other countries in HPV vaccination with the strategic implementation of campaigns not only in schools but also in facility and community settings to capture eligible girls who were not in the school systems and to reduce logistic difficulties and high costs of a purely school-based approach.[584] High costs were a barrier in the earlier stages of HPV vaccine availability, as a study found that in a survey of 147 Kenyan women, the high cost of the vaccine was met with an unwillingness to pay for it.[585]

A case-control study was conducted in Tanzania within a cluster-RCT phase of an HPV vaccination campaign of 134 primary schools, which identified the reasons for not receiving the vaccine.[586] A main reason for refusing vaccination was concerns about side effects and infertility, which was associated with being absent from school, first hearing about the HPV vaccine from a non-project source, not attending a school meeting to discuss the HPV vaccine, not having been treated by the deworming program, not knowing the location of the cervix, and not knowing that the HPV vaccine is used to prevent cervical cancer.[586] This study also highlighted the need for sensitization messages and retention of knowledge and parent meetings as critical for HPV vaccine acceptance.[586]

Conclusion

The first HPV vaccine became commercially available in 2006, and the first nationwide vaccine rollout in Africa began in 2011, with the cost per dose being negotiated in 2013 to support African countries. Following an accelerated vaccine program in 2016 for girls ages 9 to 14 in 27 countries, HPV prevalence, and cervical cancer incidence and mortality decreased. The success of the HPV campaign in Rwanda can be attributed to five key lessons. First, a robust partnership with relevant external organizations facilitated vaccine accessibility, capacity-building, rollout and implementation, sustainability, information sharing, and funding opportunities. Second, Rwanda's grade-based vaccine approach worked better than the age-based strategy because of exceptionally high school enrolment rates. It removed the challenge of establishing girls' ages, and the classrooms helped obtain consent for vaccination, spread knowledge, and decrease misconceptions through education, family planning, and hygiene awareness. Third, strong political will and leadership engagement were crucial in influencing vaccine acceptance as they secured champions and external partnerships, engaged involved parties, promoted synthesis of scientific evidence, and diffused effective communication strategies. Fourth, an intersectoral collaboration between formally appointed leaders, champions, and external change agents leveraged all of Rwanda's assets through information sharing on resources and service delivery systems, establishing clear governance structures, engaging women's groups, increasing dialogue about the vaccine, and using human resources. Finally, the varied nature of the HPV rollout sensitization and communication, along with the catch-up campaign, the strategy to reach the out-of-school target population, and multiple communication channels, targets, involved parties, and end users, were vital to the campaign's success.

12
Where We Go from Here: Translating Evidence into Policy

An ounce of prevention is worth a pound of cure.

– Benjamin Franklin, 1736

The eradication of smallpox was seen as one of the most outstanding public health achievements of the twentieth century. The burden of the disease had an intense impact on a global scale. For example, in 1959, smallpox remained endemic in 59 countries containing about 60% of the world's population. However, by 1977, the last endemic smallpox case was recorded in Somalia. By May 1980, after two years of surveillance, the World Health Assembly declared that smallpox was the first disease to have been eradicated. How did public health officials, clinicians, and other parties eradicate smallpox? The answer primarily lies in how the smallpox vaccines were implemented. The WHO relied on national campaigns and cross-sectional collaboration with federal governments to eradicate smallpox successfully.

The gap between scientifically proven health interventions and their successful implementation in the real world has historically persisted in various contexts. This gap is often within the global public health field, where public health officials know what they have to do, but they don't know how to do it.

Although the WHO launched a global campaign to eradicate smallpox in 1959, smallpox remained endemic in Africa, Asia, and South America in 1966[587] because of significant challenges encountered during the program, such as lack of funds and personnel and insufficient vaccine donations.[587] However, the eradication program was intensified in 1967, which marked a turning point. A higher-quality freeze-dried vaccine was produced in laboratories across multiple countries to address vaccine insufficiency.[587,588] In addition to mass vaccination campaigns, a case surveillance system was established, and the development of the bifurcated needle and Ped-O-Jet injector gun greatly improved vaccination procedures. According to Breman,[589] the bifurcated needle technique is simple, and almost anyone can learn it in a few minutes. By 1977, smallpox was eradicated in Africa.[587] The adoption of a strategy to achieve herd immunity was effective in eradicating smallpox in Africa. At least 80% of the population received the smallpox vaccine. Another significant innovation was developing a case surveillance system, which determines the number of cases in particular areas.[587] Using experts as operational officers contributed to the success of the smallpox vaccination program. These officers were conversant in epidemiology and control and experts in logistics, communications, and vaccine transport and storage.[589]

Several biological reasons favoured the eradication of smallpox; the most critical reasons were that recurrent infectivity did not occur, there was no animal vector, and effective and durable vaccines were available.[590] Furthermore, successful smallpox eradication placed an increased emphasis on community involvement. Such community involvement included educating locals and village chiefs about disease prevention methods and highlighting the need for early identification and treatment.[591]

The smallpox eradication program was highly feasible as it garnered cross-sectional collaboration from government officials, clinicians, and other involved parties. It had a relatively favourable cost-benefit ratio of attempting and then achieving eradication. This large cost-benefit ratio was probably the greatest global public investment in human history.

Since 1980, the eradication of smallpox has saved millions of lives. According to Dr. Donald Henderson, who led the global smallpox eradication campaign, smallpox killed at least half a billion people in the last 100 years of its existence.[592] Research has shown that about 5 million lives have been saved each year through its eradication.[593] Therefore, about 205 million lives were saved globally between 1980 and 2021.

The upfront cost of achieving eradication was USD 298 million in the 1970s.[594] At first, the initial campaign suffered from a lack of funds, resources, and political commitment, and a shortage of vaccine donations.[595] However, increased international cooperation subsequently improved, which enhanced implementation.

A more recent success is the new Ebola vaccine, a recombinant, replication-competent, vesicular stomatitis virus-based vaccine expressing the glycoprotein of a Zaire Ebolavirus (rVSV-ZEBOV). After the 2013–16 outbreak, in 2017, the USAID funded USD 20 million for the first deliveries of licensed Ebola vaccines to the GAVI-funded global emergency

Ebola vaccine stockpile for future outbreaks. In 2021, Merck entered into an agreement with UNICEF to create the world's first global stockpile of the vaccine, with more than 500,000 doses in the stockpile as of March 2023.[596] This vaccine was also included in the GAVI-funded stockpile, with other candidate vaccines for Ebola from that year that were in different developmental stages eligible for inclusion in the stockpile upon the WHO prequalification.

GAVI used an innovative financing mechanism, the advance purchase commitment, to incentivize manufactures to speed up Ebola vaccine development, so it could procure the doses, with the agreement being the first of its kind. The commitment allowed investigational vaccines to be deployed for compassionate use during outbreaks, before the vaccines were licensed. In addition, access to the stockpile was free for GAVI-eligible low- and lower-middle-income countries, and they were provided support for operational costs relating to outbreak response immunization activities. As a result of the joint efforts of various organizations, like GAVI, the WHO, and UNICEF, a large number of people were vaccinated against Ebola during the 2018 outbreak in the Democratic Republic of the Congo.[597] Since the West African clinical trials, the rVSV-ZEBOV vaccine was first deployed during the April–July 2018 Ebola outbreak in the Democratic Republic of the Congo.[598] Ebola emerged in the country in April 2018[599] and an outbreak was declared on May 8, followed by contact tracing and ring vaccination two weeks later. Ring vaccination reduced the area at risk by 70.4% and the level of risk by 70.1%, with a projected reduction of risk of 54.2%, 76.8%, and 85.0% in three populous urban centres within a month.[600] Compared with the West Africa outbreak, this outbreak was controlled quickly,[601] owing to swift vaccine deployment. If the campaign was delayed by a week, risk reduction was projected to drop from 70.4% to 33.3%, relative to no vaccination.[598]

In 2019, over 111,000 people had been vaccinated in the Democratic Republic of the Congo since the 2018 outbreak, but despite the highly efficacious vaccine, cases were rising, largely owing to critical security incidents. Consequently, the WHO's Strategic Advisory Group of Experts issued new recommendations that included using pop-up and targeted geographic vaccination, accelerating the vaccination process, adjusting dosage, expanding the eligible population for the vaccine, introducing more experimental vaccines, and training healthcare personnel and medical students. Pop-up and targeted geographic vaccination were previously successful in the field by the WHO in making the ring vaccination process quicker, more secure, and responsive to community feedback.[602] These approaches had already been successfully implemented to address security concerns and tensions within the community. In the case of rVSV-ZEBOV, vaccines were recommended to be administered in temporary, protected vaccination sites, instead of being set up at the residences of contacts. Those with reported cases of Ebola, and the contacts of their contacts, in a particular area, would be invited for vaccination at these sites. The sites would offer security to the medical teams, allow them to vaccinate more cases, especially in areas without vaccination rings, and help reduce stigma for those seeking treatment.[603]

Health Systems, Funding and Scaling Up in Africa

Financing is one of the building blocks of a health system. Financing is needed to use evidence-based planning and mobilize budget consumption and ensure the implementation of a cost-effective intervention. Additional components of a health system include service delivery, health workforce, information, medical products/vaccines/technology, financing, and leadership/governments.

Health systems funding in Africa is an accumulation of finances from the Ministry of Health, multilateral and bilateral agencies, NGOs, and foundations. According to the WHO Global Health Expenditure database, in 2019, sub-Saharan Africa's health expenditure was 4.97% of its GDP. This percentage expenditure is very low compared with high-income nations, such as Canada and the United States, which spent 10.84% and 16.77%, respectively, of their GDP on healthcare services in 2019.[604] Healthcare expenditure plays a critical role in improving health outcomes by increasing life expectancy, reducing mortality rates, and lowering infant deaths.[605] In regions of Africa, various health system approaches are used, including pyramidal healthcare, community medicine, and other complex structures.[606] For example, in Tanzania, thousands of village health facilities are placed throughout the country to provide basic preventative and primary healthcare, although the medical teams are limited and sometimes under-trained.[606] In Uganda, village health teams and volunteer community health workers provide health advice to patients and refer complex cases to health facilities.[606] In this approach, it is common for patients to be transferred from facility to facility; the health facilities are understaffed and have inadequate funding. High-income residents depend highly on private insurance, whereas low-income residents depend on public clinics.[606]

In Africa, user fees are a significant issue because of low benefits for in-patient care, lack of transparency, and inadequate national health insurance funding.[606] Implementing various interventions is challenging because of limited numbers of trained healthcare professionals and implementation science experts. Many research projects and health interventions have been organized in Africa; however, the research-policy gap remains an issue.[607] There is a need to scale up healthcare interventions and technologies through adequate funding.

The WHO reported in 2021 that most healthcare spending is invested in infectious disease treatment in LMIC, and 63% of those countries are in Africa.[608] The World Bank invested over USD 39 billion in Africa for the COVID-19 pandemic response.[609] It also reported that sub-Saharan Africa's current health expenditure per capita is approximately USD 83.[610] The International Monetary Fund loan acceptance is also used in various regions of Africa, and this has led to a rise in the price of imported drugs and medical equipment.[606] In 2022, approximately USD 1.65 billion was invested in health through all-cause development assistance for health in North Africa.[611] In that same year, approximately USD 15.4 billion was invested in health through all-cause development assistance for health in sub-Saharan Africa.[611]

Funds that are aimed directly towards scaling up health in Africa are limited. In addition, there are a few examples that illustrate the financial burden of this process. Sub-Saharan Africa has the greatest HIV/AIDS burden worldwide, and in 2016, only USD 4.5 billion was invested in scaling up HIV/AIDS interventions, however, an annual addition of USD 7 billion is still needed.[612] Many multilateral and bilateral agencies invest in health research in Africa. The US National Institutes of Health constitutes approximately 64% of global research funding in Africa.[37]

Welcome Trust and UK Medical Research Council contribute approximately 13% and 12%, respectively, to global health research in Africa.[37] Other agencies such as the European Union, the Canada Institutes of Health Research, the European and Developing Countries Clinical Trials Partnership, the Swedish International Development Cooperation Agency, and the Swedish Research Council each contribute between 1% and 3% of global health research funding in Africa.[37] NGOs and foundations, such as the Bill and Melinda Gates Foundation, also invest in Africa.

Healthcare expenditure has been low over the years in developing regions of the world, particularly in African countries, compared with developed countries such as the United Kingdom, Canada, and United States. In 2019, sub-Saharan Africa spent only USD 79.43 per capita on healthcare, compared with the Middle East and North Africa, which spent USD 512.76 per capita, and Latin America and the Caribbean, which spent USD 662.04 per capita on healthcare.[613]

The data from the WHO on health expenditure per capita for the year 2019 indicates that in sub-Saharan Africa, Madagascar spent the lowest amount (USD 19.85), while Seychelles spent the highest (USD 839.77). In Latin America and the Caribbean, Haiti spent the lowest (USD 56.99), and the Bahamas spent the highest (USD 2004). In South Asia, Pakistan spent about USD 39.50 on healthcare.[610]

Furthermore, according to the UNESCO Institutes of Statistics, in 2021, only 0.33% of sub-Saharan Africa's GDP was spent on research and development. South Asia spent 0.57%, Latin America and the Caribbean spent 0.55%, and North America and Western Europe spent 2.93%.[614]

Nevertheless, several international organizations have funded implementation science research in Africa. These include the Welcome Trust, the American Society for Clinical Pathology, the Bill and Melinda Gates Foundation, and the Coalition for Research in Global Oncology (CIRGO). In 2020, CIRGO awarded USD 480,000 in capacity-building grants to support eight implementation science research projects in Africa. Each project received a USD 60,000 grant to create country-specific initiatives focusing on increasing early detection of breast cancer, improving cancer data quality, enhancing rural access to cancer testing and diagnostic services, and strengthening cancer registries.[615,616]

Increasing primary healthcare in Africa's health systems could provide the opportunity to scale up health interventions and accelerate the health system's progress towards SDGs.[606]

Considerations

1. Thrive on Tension for Change in Initiating and Sustaining Health Innovations

Tension for change exists where there is dissatisfaction with the status quo. The construct *tension for change* is part of the inner setting domain of the CFIR that relates to the characteristics of the implementing organization and its partners, which might influence implementation.[250] For example, a year before the highly successful HPV campaign, in 2010, Rwanda experienced 986 cases of cervical cancer, with 678 women dying from the disease. In 2011, Rwanda implemented its national HPV vaccination program and achieved 93% coverage of eligible girls, the highest coverage in the world. There was tension for change, which Rwanda's Ministry of Health capitalized on by collaborating with Merck to provide the Gardasil HPV vaccine to all girls of the appropriate age. By 2011, Rwanda had become the first African country to launch an HPV vaccination campaign, providing vaccines to all 12-year-old female students. It is difficult to create tension for change when none exists, but where it does, as described for the meningitis vaccine project (Chapter 10) and the HPV project (Chapter 11), it can be capitalized on to initiate or sustain scale-up of the innovations.

2. Leverage the Commitment from Governments for Sustainable Scale

Federal or state governments have a great influence on how innovations scale through their authority and influence within the health systems. The cases covered in this book, from VAS programs to the MomConnect mHealth initiative, depend strongly on government influence. Therefore, the government must prioritize the scaling up of evidence-based innovations and its financial commitment to them. In addition, innovators and external partners wanting to see innovations scale in the country must liaise and draw on the resources and goodwill of government ministries or parastatals. Several processes might include incorporating these health innovations into healthcare systems and budget allocation through the availability of required personnel, as was evident in several malaria bed net programs.

3. Provide Adequate Resources

Adequate resources are required to scale evidence-based innovations effectively. These resources include funding, human resources, and materials or equipment needed for activities and their implementation. The associated CFIR construct *available resources* relates to the implementation and ongoing operations, including money, training, education, physical space, and time.[248] Among existing innovations studied, the most significant barrier has probably been inadequate funding, which is critical for resource-constrained settings.

4. Build on Trust

In the context of global health innovations, trust operates on four planes: partnership, government, technology, and community.[617] Although all four are significant, trust in innovation seems to be a limiting factor. To improve the uptake of any innovation, users must trust it. The *intervention characteristics* of the CFIR is most related to the technology trust. In the Theoretical Domains Framework, the domain *knowledge* relates to the awareness of the intervention and its scientific rationale. The issue of trust has been a pronounced challenge because of a multitude of factors for biotech crops. There has been great distrust at multiple levels, including the development of regulation, interest by the private sector, and distrust of promises, delivery, and much more. Innovations should focus on trust from the perspective of beneficiaries – moving towards a trust-centred paradigm.

5. *Provide Adequate Training Capacity*

A significant gap in the scale-up of most health innovations is human resource capacity as it relates to high staff turnover, inadequacy, and lack of training. One of the bottlenecks in implementation is training. In Africa, as shown by the capacity in implementation, this is consistently cited as a significant barrier in the praziquantel administration, VAS, and even mHealth programs. Access to knowledge and information under the CFIR domain best captures the training issue: ease of access to digestible information and knowledge about the intervention and how to incorporate it into work tasks. Training is one of the best approaches to accessing knowledge and information. The critical success of the NTD program in Ghana was a result of the extensive training provided to all personnel involved in the MDA process. One month before the MDA program, the NTDP held a national workshop to train the trainers, which brought together deputy directors of public health, regional disease control officers, and regional NTDP coordinators, as well as regional School Health Education Program (SHEP) coordinators from the Ghana Education Service (GES). Following the adaptation of the training curriculum by the NTD program , regional and district-level training were held for district health directors, district SHEP coordinators, district disease control officers, head teachers, school health education coordinators, and GES circuit supervisors.

6. *Foster Multisectoral Coordination in the Scale of Innovations*

To effectively scale up evidence-based innovations, multisectoral and international coordination must be improved. A coordinated effort by various sectors, including the ministries of health and education, NGOs, and international organizations, is required. Leveraging the strengths and diverse approaches of the sectors can eliminate policy implementation barriers and facilitate scale-up efforts. Coordination across government ministries, for example, is critical for identifying sector intersections and opportunities for collaborative planning. In Rwanda, for instance, Social Determinants of Health are addressed through multisectoral action. The government created four ministerial clusters to maximize intersectoral collaboration: the social cluster, the economic cluster, the governance cluster, and the justice cluster. Such clusters enhance intersectoral consultations and collaboration, which was evident in the HPV project.

7. Focus Efforts on Innovations That Are Evidence Based

Governments and organizations should focus energy and effort on evidence-based innovations that have been tested and validated to save and improve lives. Time, effort, and resources that the government and private sectors spend on the scale-up of innovations that have no proof of concept can be a significant opportunity cost. Instead, the investment needs to be in evidence-based innovations that have demonstrated proof of concept. Evidence-based innovations help to curb expenditure and improve healthcare.

8. Create Policies, Incentives, and Structures That Allow for Scale

There should be supportive policies and frameworks to scale up evidence-based innovations. Policies involve rules, regulations, guidelines, and administrative standards used by governments to translate national laws and policies into programs and services. A favourable policy environment will facilitate the scale-up of health interventions. Having supportive policies and legislation for implementation encourages collaboration and increases the scalability and sustainability of interventions. For example, the MomConnect initiative faced few integration barriers because of the National Health Normative Standards Framework for Interoperability in mHealth in South Africa.

9. Communicate, Communicate, Communicate

To effectively scale up the innovations, clear communication and understanding of the importance and benefits of evidence-based innovation are required among all groups involved in the implementation process and the beneficiaries. A significant barrier to the scale uptake of evidence-based innovation is a lack of knowledge of its importance and the potential for false information and myths to flourish around the interventions. This was the case for polio vaccination programs. Therefore, efforts must be made to communicate and engage with beneficiaries to increase acceptance of the innovation. In Nigeria's case with the praziquantel MDA program, the primary barrier to the acceptance of the drug was the spread of misinformation through a lack of awareness and misconception about praziquantel.

10. Focus on Champions

Champions are characterized by their willingness to risk their informal status and reputation because they believe so strongly in the intervention. Champions actively support the intervention during its implementation. Champions are critical facilitators that can effectively scale up evidence-based innovations and influence the decisions of communities. Identifying these champions and engaging with them can effectively scale up evidence-based innovations. In the case of HPV vaccination implementation in Rwanda, Rwanda's First Lady, H. E. Jeannette Kagame, was a key champion. In the MomConnect program, the minister of health was a key champion. Both were instrumental in the immensely successful scale-up of the respective innovations.

Discussion Questions

1. They Came, They Saw, They Scaled: Health Innovations for Impact

1 What are some barriers to implementing and sustaining evidence-based health innovations in Africa? Use two African countries as case studies to illustrate these challenges.
2 Summarize the five points of the teaching tool that Curran[13] developed to help individuals think like implementation scientists, using a specific health innovation as an example.
3 How does implementation science bridge the gap between health research findings and real-world practice? Detail the six critical areas of implementation science frameworks and their role in addressing the delivery gap.
4 What is grand convergence, and how does it aim to bridge health disparities between high-income countries and LMICs? What interventions or strategies could aid Africa in achieving grand convergence?
5 How can the success story of malaria bed net adoption in Tanzania act as a model for other health innovations in Africa?
6 Why is there a notable disparity in research and development investments between Western and African nations? How can African governments and organizations incentivize investment in research and innovation?
7 How have African countries demonstrated their innovation and implementation capacities despite their diverse challenges?
8 Provide examples when a lack of effective implementation or scale-up prevented a potential health solution from reaching its intended beneficiaries.

9 In what ways do local culture and regional constraints influence the effectiveness of universally recognized health strategies?
10 How can collaborative efforts and pan-African initiatives enhance the scale-up of health innovations in Africa?
11 What are the ethical considerations when introducing and scaling health innovations in LMICs?

2. The ORS Paradox: Why the Gap and What to Do about It

1 How have various iterations of ORS been influenced by advancements in medical knowledge over the decades?
2 What roles have international organizations like UNICEF, the WHO, and USAID played in promoting ORS in Africa?
3 What are the primary challenges and facilitators in ensuring ORS reaches those most in need in Africa?
4 How have different African regions, like Sierra Leone and Mali, adopted nation-specific strategies for ORS implementation, and what lessons can we learn from them?
5 How have countries like Egypt ensured the continuous supply and distribution of ORS across both urban and rural areas?
6 In what ways have public health campaigns and mass media been used to increase the knowledge and understanding of ORS in various communities?
7 How have design considerations, like packaging and taste, influenced the acceptance and uptake of ORS in different communities?
8 What are some innovative solutions that might bridge the delivery gap of ORS to children who need it?
9 What are some potential drawbacks or concerns associated with widespread ORS distribution and use?
10 What roles have local governments, regulatory bodies, and the public and private sectors played in the scale-up of ORS in Africa?

3. Handwashing and Hygiene: Basic but Crucial

1 Why is handwashing compliance unequal across countries in Africa?
2 How did the shift from miasma theory to germ theory influence the evolution of handwashing awareness and practices? How did historical figures like Ignaz Philipp Semmelweis and Florence Nightingale contribute to this evolution?

3 How have global health organizations like the CDC and WHO influenced handwashing practices over the decades?
4 Discuss the significance of initiatives like the Save Lives: Clean Your Hands Initiative and Water, Sanitation, and Hygiene (WASH) program. How have they impacted global handwashing awareness and practices?
5 How do handwashing practices in clinical settings, like hospitals and healthcare facilities, differ from those in community settings? What strategies have been used to scale handwashing in both settings?
6 How effective are grassroots initiatives like the Tippy Tap technology and Social Art for Behaviour Change in promoting and sustaining handwashing habits in local communities?
7 What role does the economic factor play in the implementation and success of handwashing programs, especially in resource-constrained settings?
8 How have global events, such as the COVID-19 pandemic, influenced the urgency and methods of promoting hand hygiene?
9 How do cultural or societal factors in certain African countries influence the acceptance and adherence to handwashing practices?
10 How can innovations, both in technology and in strategy, be scaled up to ensure a more significant impact in promoting handwashing practices across different settings and regions?
11 Discuss the role of local leadership and community engagement in the success of handwashing interventions. How can these be optimized for greater impact?

4. Neglected Tropical Diseases Innovations: The Forgotten

1 How does praziquantel address various neglected tropical diseases?
2 Why do you think it is hard to scale up implementation of praziquantel across Africa?
3 In what ways do partnerships between research institutions, governments, and pharmaceutical companies contribute to the development and scaling of innovative solutions for NTDs in Africa?
4 How do community-based and participatory approaches play a role in the design and implementation of innovative interventions for NTDs, and what are the key considerations for ensuring community acceptance and sustainability?

5 How well can the distribution of praziquantel be adapted to fit different contexts and cultures across Africa, aside from countries discussed in this chapter?
6 What role can education and awareness campaigns play in promoting the adoption of innovative solutions for NTDs, and how can culturally sensitive communication strategies be developed?
7 How can innovations in drug development and distribution contribute to more cost-effective and accessible treatments for NTDs in resource-limited settings?
8 How can governments and international organizations support the scale-up of successful NTD innovations, and what policy frameworks are needed to ensure sustained impact?
9 What role does cross-disciplinary collaboration play in driving innovation for NTDs in Africa, and how can lessons from successful collaborations be applied to future initiatives?
10 If you were a WHO employee working with a national government in [a country of your choice] and wanted to urge them to spend more funding for the MDA of praziquantel, what evidence would you show them and what would you advise them to do?
11 What are some barriers to implementing large-scale praziquantel programs in Africa?
12 What role do rumours and misinformation play in successfully implementing a treatment, such as praziquantel, to a target population? If you were tasked to work with a local government to address rumours of a particular medication causing death for children, what would you do?

5. Biotech Crops: To Trust or Not to Trust

1 How are biotech crops an evidence-based intervention to address food security in Africa?
2 What was the first country in Africa to begin biotech crop ventures?
3 What was the impact from the first few countries to begin biotech crop ventures in other African countries?
4 Using any two countries mentioned in this chapter, how were biotech crop innovations adapted from one country to another, considering the different context between the two countries?
5 How do biotech crops contribute to food security in Africa, and what challenges do they pose in terms of access and distribution?

6 Pick one country discussed in this chapter, and describe how it improved the uptake of a particular biotech crop innovation.
7 How does the adoption of biotech crops in Africa impact traditional farming practices and agricultural knowledge?
8 What ethical considerations should be taken into account when promoting biotech crops in Africa, especially in relation to cultural values?
9 What roles do you think trust plays in the successful adoption of biotech crops in Africa?
10 What methods would you take to build trust towards biotech implementation?
11 How do you think local communities should be actively involved in the decision-making processes related to the introduction of biotech crops, and how does community engagement contribute to building trust?
12 How can biotech companies collaborate with local farmers and agricultural communities to address concerns and build mutual trust, considering the potential impact on traditional farming practices?
13 What regulatory frameworks and oversight mechanisms can be put in place to build trust in the safety and ethical considerations surrounding biotech crops in Africa? (Hint: Consider forming councils and local advisory groups or creating a diverse team to capture all perspectives.)
14 In what ways do biotech crops affect the livelihoods of smallhold farmers in Africa, and what policies could be implemented to support their integration?

6. Vitamin A Has a Story to Tell

1 When was vitamin A first discovered as an important micronutrient playing a significant role in our overall health?
2 How does VAS impact the nutritional status of vulnerable populations, such as pregnant women and young children, and what are the potential long-term effects on community health?
3 What are the specific health challenges related to VAD in Africa, and how does supplementation address these issues?
4 How does VAS contribute to improving maternal and child health outcomes in African communities, and what evidence supports its efficacy?
5 What role does vitamin A play in boosting the immune system, and how does supplementation impact the overall health

resilience of populations in Africa, particularly in the context of infectious diseases, such as measles?

6 In what ways can VAS be adapted to various contexts and cultures in Africa?

7 How does the success of VAS programs in Africa depend on community participation and awareness, and what approaches can be used to effectively engage local communities?

8 Choose any country discussed in this chapter and describe any cultural or social factors that influence the acceptance and adherence to VAS. How can these factors be addressed in program design to increase the use of VAS?

9 How much does it cost to create VAS?

10 What are the economic implications of VAS, both in terms of healthcare costs and productivity gains, and how do these factors contribute to sustainable development?

11 How can international collaborations and partnerships enhance the effectiveness of VAS programs in Africa, and what lessons can be learned from successful collaborations in this chapter?

7. mHealth: Spreading or Stalling?

1 In what way do mHealth initiatives impact maternal health?

2 When did mHealth initiatives begin to be implemented?

3 What factors contribute to the successful scale-up of mHealth initiatives in Africa?

4 How does the level of community engagement and participation influence the scalability of mHealth initiatives, and what strategies can be employed to enhance community involvement?

5 What role do technological infrastructure and connectivity play in the success or failure of scaling up mHealth initiatives, and how can challenges related to access be effectively addressed?

6 How do cultural and social factors impact the adoption and sustainability of mHealth initiatives, and what cultural competency strategies are essential for successful scale-up?

7 In what ways can partnerships between governments, private sectors, and NGOs contribute to the scalability of mHealth initiatives, and what challenges need to be overcome in forming and maintaining these collaborations?

8 What role does user acceptance and behaviour change play in the success of mHealth initiatives, and how can design and implementation strategies be tailored to meet the needs and preferences of diverse user groups?

9 How can lessons from successful mHealth initiatives discussed in this chapter be applied to improve the scalability of future projects, and what are the key transferable elements that contribute to success?
10 How do issues of privacy, data security, and ethical considerations impact the scale-up of mHealth initiatives?

8. Malaria Bed Nets: A Prism of Implementation Complexity

1 When were bed nets first developed?
2 How are bed nets effective at decreasing the transmission of malaria?
3 When were bed nets first introduced to Africa as a mechanism to decrease the transmission of malaria?
4 What are the key challenges and successes in the implementation of bed net distribution programs to combat malaria in different regions of Africa?
5 How does the adaptability of bed net distribution programs vary across urban and rural areas, and what strategies can be employed to ensure equitable access in both settings?
6 How can partnerships between governments, non-profit organizations, and the private sector contribute to the successful scale-up of bed net distribution programs in Africa?
7 How do cultural beliefs and practices influence the acceptance and use of bed nets, and what culturally sensitive approaches can be implemented to enhance their effectiveness?
8 What role does community engagement play in the successful implementation and scale-up of bed net distribution, and how can community participation be maximized?
9 How do environmental factors, such as climate and geography, impact the effectiveness of bed nets in different regions of Africa, and how can these factors be taken into account in implementation strategies?
10 How can education and awareness campaigns be tailored to address misconceptions and promote the proper use of bed nets?
11 How can lessons learned from successful bed net implementation in one African country discussed in this chapter be applied to facilitate the scale-up of similar programs in other countries, and what key contextual differences need to be considered?

9. Polio Eradication: Are We There Yet?

1 What factors contributed to the resurgence of the poliovirus in Africa after it was declared polio free in 2020?

2 Compare and contrast the inactive poliovirus (IPV) vaccine and oral poliovirus vaccine (OPV). Why do you think OPV is still used in other countries, even though it is discontinued in the United States?
3 What role do community leaders and religious scholars play in influencing people's decision to accept or reject the polio vaccine?
4 Identify and explain the communication strategies that can be used to effectively address rumours and misinformation about vaccines?
5 What impact did the infrastructure in African countries have on the success or failure of polio vaccination campaigns?
6 How do cultural beliefs shape public perception and acceptance of the polio vaccine?
7 In what ways was the delivery of vaccination campaigns adapted to local context and challenges in Africa?
8 Discuss how global organizations and international partnerships drove polio eradication efforts, and identify any barriers or facilitators they encountered.
9 How did the intervention design of polio vaccination campaigns affect public acceptance and coverage?
10 Drawing from the experiences in Africa, how can global health organizations better prepare for vaccine hesitancy or refusal in future public health crises?

10. The Meningitis Vaccine Project: Remaking an Implementation Climate

1 How did the MenAfricaVac vaccine change the landscape of meningitis A epidemics in the Meningitis Belt of Africa?
2 How did the collaboration between organizations like PATH, the WHO, and the Serum Institute of India influence the success of the MenAfriVac vaccine?
3 Discuss the significance of the initial funding and support from the Bill and Melinda Gates Foundation for the MVP in facilitating its progress and success.
4 Explain how the MVP was able to produce the MenAfriVac vaccine for under USD 0.50 per dose and how this affected the vaccine's affordability and adoption in Africa.
5 Describe how the leadership efforts of Dr. Marc Laforce, along with other African leaders, drove the MVP forward?
6 What roles did the public and private sectors play in the success of the MVP?

7 Since the MenAfriVac vaccine mainly targets meningitis serotype A, what challenges does Africa still face in addressing other serotypes of meningococcal meningitis?
8 Briefly describe the four key lessons learned from the MVP. How can these lessons be leveraged for future health initiatives in Africa?
9 What key attributes made the MenAfriVac vaccine uniquely suited to meet the challenges of meningitis serotype A in Africa?
10 Given the impact of the COVID-19 pandemic on vaccination campaigns, what strategies can ensure the continued success of the MenAfriVac vaccine and other health campaigns in Africa?
11 How did the success of the MenAfriVac vaccine impact health policies and strategies related to infectious disease control in Africa?
12 How was the MVP able to maintain a unified vision and momentum despite having a large and diverse group of partners and involved parties?

11. Human Papillomavirus Campaign: A Success Story in Rwanda

1 How did the initial high cost of the HPV vaccine impede its rollout in LMICs, especially in Africa?
2 What made Rwanda's grade-based vaccination strategy more successful (in the context of its HPV vaccination campaigns) than the WHO recommended age-based strategy?
3 What major barriers emerged regarding HPV vaccine sensitization and communication during its implementation?
4 How did strong political will and leadership engagement in Rwanda contribute to the success of the HPV vaccine campaign?
5 Describe the factors that contributed to the high prevalence of cervical cancer in sub-Saharan Africa, relative to global rates.
6 What role did the intersectoral collaboration strategy of Rwanda's HPV campaign play in fostering community trust and vaccine uptake?
7 Identify potential challenges other African countries might face when attempting to replicate Rwanda's HPV vaccine campaign, given their unique sociopolitical landscapes.
8 Explain how Rwanda's external partnerships shaped the broader African perspective on the significance of international collaborations in public health efforts, and how these partnerships supported HPV vaccine campaigns in Africa.
9 How can future health campaigns in Africa apply the lessons learned from Rwanda to achieve better outcomes?

10 What influence have cultural, social, and economic factors had on HPV vaccine acceptance and hesitancy in Africa, and what strategies can be adopted to address these factors?
11 What might be the benefits of integrating health education along with HPV vaccinations in schools?
12 What are some ways for African countries to ensure they sustain the momentum and success of HPV vaccine campaigns?

12. Where We Go from Here: Translating Evidence into Policy

1 What efforts led to the global eradication of smallpox after the WHO's attempt in 1959?
2 What characteristics of the advance purchase commitment made it an innovative agreement, and how did it support vaccination against Ebola in Africa?
3 Compare and contrast the eradication strategies for smallpox and Ebola, as well as their successes and challenges.
4 What are the advantages and disadvantages of the different healthcare systems in Africa, in terms of preventing and treating infectious diseases?
5 How does funding play a role in the scale-up and success of health interventions in Africa?
6 How can tension for change be capitalized on to initiate or sustain health innovations in Africa?
7 Identify the four planes of trust and provide examples of how each can either impede or facilitate implementation of health interventions in Africa.
8 Map out three CFIR domains to any of the 10 considerations provided in this chapter.
9 What is the significance of multisectoral collaborations and partnerships in scaling-up health interventions in Africa, and how can these partnerships contribute to closing the research-policy gap in Africa?
10 Choose one infectious disease and apply each of the 10 considerations shared in this chapter to create a successful health intervention strategy.
11 What might be the advantages of leveraging champions to support a health intervention, compared with the government or health organizations?

References

1 Ezezika, O., & Singer, P. A. (2010). Genetically engineered oil-eating microbes for bioremediation: Prospects and regulatory challenges. *Technology in Society*, *32*(4), 331–335. https://doi.org/10.1016/j.techsoc.2010.10.010

2 Kimble, L., & Massoud, R. (2017). What do we mean by innovation in healthcare. *European Medical Journal*, *1*(1), 89–91.

3 Bhargava, K., & Bhargava, D. (2007). Evidence based health care. *Sultan Qaboos University Medical Journal*, *7*(2), 105–107. Medline:21748091

4 Santo, K., & Redfern, J. (2020). Digital health innovations to improve cardiovascular disease care. *Current Atherosclerosis Reports*, *22*(12), 71. https://doi.org/10.1007/s11883-020-00889-x. Medline:33009975

5 Pillay, Y., & Motsoaledi, P. A. (2018). Digital health in South Africa: Innovating to improve health. *BMJ Global Health*, *3*(Suppl. 2), Article e000722. https://doi.org/10.1136/bmjgh-2018-000722. Medline:29713513

6 Leonard, E., de Kock, I., & Bam, W. (2020). Barriers and facilitators to implementing evidence-based health innovations in low- and middle-income countries: A systematic literature review. *Evaluation and Program Planning*, *82*, 101832. https://doi.org/10.1016/j.evalprogplan.2020.101832. Medline:32585317

7 Motiwala, F., & Ezezika, O. (2021). Barriers to scaling health technologies in sub-Saharan Africa: Lessons from Ethiopia, Nigeria, and Rwanda. *African Journal of Science, Technology, Innovation and Development*, *14*(7), 1–10. https://doi.org/10.1080/20421338.2021.1985203

8 Al-Bader, S., Daar, A. S., & Singer, P. A. (2010). Science-based health innovation in Ghana: Health entrepreneurs point the way to a new development path. *BMC International Health and Human Rights*, *10*(1), S2. https://doi.org/10.1186/1472-698X-10-S1-S2. Medline:21144073

9 Kamunyori, S., Al-Bader, S., Sewankambo, N., Singer, P. A., & Daar, A. S. (2010). Science-based health innovation in Uganda: Creative strategies for applying research to development. *BMC International Health and*

Human Rights, 10(1), S5. https://doi.org/10.1186/1472-698X-10-S1-S5. Medline:21144076

10 World Health Organization. (2016). *Scaling up projects and initiatives for better health: From concepts to practice.* https://iris.who.int/bitstream/handle/10665/343809/9789289051552-eng.pdf

11 Billings, D. L., Crane, B. B., Benson, J., Solo, J., & Fetters, T. (2007). Scaling-up a public health innovation: A comparative study of post-abortion care in Bolivia and Mexico. *Social Science & Medicine (1982), 64*(11), 2210–2222. https://doi.org/10.1016/j.socscimed.2007.02.026. Medline:17408826

12 Foege, W. H. (2011). *House on fire: The fight to eradicate smallpox*. University of California Press.

13 Curran, G. M. (2020). Implementation science made too simple: A teaching tool. *Implementation Science Communications, 1*(1), 27. https://doi.org/10.1186/s43058-020-00001-z. Medline:32885186

14 Munos, M. K., Walker, C. L. F., & Black, R. E. (2010). The effect of oral rehydration solution and recommended home fluids on diarrhoea mortality. *International Journal of Epidemiology, 39*(Suppl. 1), i75–i87. https://doi.org/10.1093/ije/dyq025. Medline:20348131

15 Dadonaite, B., Ritchie, H., & Roser, M. (2018). *Diarrheal diseases*. Our World in Data. https://ourworldindata.org/diarrheal-diseases

16 Gregorio, G. V., Gonzales, M. L. M., Dans, L. F., & Martinez, E. G. (2016). Polymer-based oral rehydration solution for treating acute watery diarrhoea. *Cochrane Library, 12*, 1–107. https://doi.org/10.1002/14651858.CD006519.pub3. Medline:27959472

17 Greenhalgh, T., & Papoutsi, C. (2019). Spreading and scaling up innovation and improvement. *BMJ, 365*, 1–8. https://doi.org/10.1136/bmj.l2068. Medline:31076440

18 Meyers, D., Durlak, J., & Wandersman, A. (2012). The Quality Implementation Framework: A synthesis of critical steps in the implementation process. *American Journal of Community Psychology, 50*(3–4), 1–20. https://doi.org/10.1007/s10464-012-9522-x. Medline:22644083

19 Blanchard, C., Livet, M., Ward, C., Sorge, L., Sorensen, T. D., & McClurg, M. R. (2017). The active implementation frameworks: A roadmap for advancing implementation of comprehensive medication management in primary care. *Research in Social and Administrative Pharmacy, 13*(5), 922–929. https://doi.org/10.1016/j.sapharm.2017.05.006. Medline:28549800

20 Nyonator, F. K., Awoonor-Williams, J. K., Phillips, J. F., Jones, T. C., & Miller, R. A. (2005). The Ghana Community-based Health Planning and Services Initiative for scaling up service delivery innovation. *Health Policy and Planning, 20*(1), 25–34. https://doi.org/10.1093/heapol/czi003. Medline:15689427

21 Barnabas, K., Yeboah, B., Letsa, T., & Mensa, E. (2020). Progress of community-based health planning and health services in Ghana. *Global Scientific Journals, 7*(12), 1212–1226.

22 Carter, M. (2015, June 1). *Many South African women become infected with HIV during pregnancy posing high risk of transmission to their infants.* Aidsmap. https://www.aidsmap.com/news/jun-2015/many-south-african-women-become-infected-hiv-during-pregnancy-posing-high-risk

23 Wagle, K. (2025, February 25). Prevention of Mother-to-Child Transmission (PMTCT) of HIV. Public Health Notes. Retrieved from https://www.publichealthnotes.com/prevention-of-mother-to-child-transmission-pmtct-of-hiv/

24 Bhardwaj, S., Barron, P., Pillay, Y., Treger-Slavin, L., Robinson, P., Goga, A., & Sherman, G. (2014). Elimination of mother-to-child transmission of HIV in South Africa: Rapid scale-up using quality improvement. *South African Medical Journal = Suid-Afrikaanse Tydskrif Vir Geneeskunde, 104*(3 Suppl. 1), 239–243. https://doi.org/10.7196/samj.7605. Medline:24893500

25 Mnyani, CN., Tait, CL., Peters, RPH., Struthers, H., Violari, A., Gray, G., Buckmann, E., Chersich, M., & McIntyre, J. (2020). Implementation of a PMTCT programme in a high HIV prevalence setting in Johannesburg, South Africa: 2002–2015. *Southern African Journal of HIV Medicine, 21*(1), 1–7. https://doi.org/10.4102/sajhivmed.v21i1.1024. Medline:32284888

26 Basinga, P., Gertler, P. J., Binagwaho, A., Soucat, A. L., Sturdy, J., & Vermeersch, C. M. (2011). Effect on maternal and child health services in Rwanda of payment to primary health-care providers for performance: An impact evaluation. *The Lancet, 377*(9775), 1421–1428. https://doi.org/10.1016/S0140-6736(11)60177-3. Medline:21515164

27 Nsanzimana, S., Prabhu, K., McDermott, H., Karita, E., Forrest, J. I., Drobac, P., Farmer, P., Mills, E. J., & Binagwaho, A. (2015). Improving health outcomes through concurrent HIV program scale-up and health system development in Rwanda: 20 years of experience. *BMC Medicine, 13*(1), 1–7. https://doi.org/10.1186/s12916-015-0443-z. Medline:26354601

28 Donovan, P. (2002). Rape and HIV/AIDS in Rwanda. *The Lancet, 360,* s17–s18. https://doi.org/10.1016/s0140-6736(02)11804-6. Medline:12504487

29 Schieber, G. J., Gottret, P., Fleisher, L. K., & Leive, A. A. (2007). Financing global health: Mission unaccomplished. *Health Affairs, 26*(4), 921–934. https://doi.org/10.1377/hlthaff.26.4.921. Medline:17630434

30 Simiyu, K., Daar, A. S., Hughes, M., & Singer, P. A. (2010). Science-based health innovation in Rwanda: Unlocking the potential of a late

bloomer. *BMC International Health and Human Rights*, *10*(1), 1–11. https://doi.org/10.1186/1472-698X-10-S1-S3. Medline:21144074

31 Watkins, S. C., Robinson, A., Dalious, M., & Initiative, I. K. (2013). *Evaluation of the information and communications technology for maternal, newborn and child health project known locally as "Chipatala Cha Pa Foni" (Health Center by Phone)*. Invest in Knowledge Initiative. https://www.villagereach.org/wp-content/uploads/2017/07/ICT_for_MNCH_Report_131211md_FINAL.pdf

32 Malanga, D. F. (2017). Implementation of mobile health initiatives in Malawi: current status, issues, and challenges. In K. Moahi, K. Bwalya, & P. Sebina (Eds.), *Health information systems and the advancement of medical practice in developing countries* (pp. 115–128). IGI Global. https://doi.org/10.4018/978-1-5225-2262-1.ch007

33 van Niekerk, L., Fosiko, N., Likaka, A., Blauvelt, C. P., Msiska, B., & Manderson, L. (2023). From idea to systems solution: Enhancing access to primary care in Malawi. *BMC Health Services Research*, *23*(1), 547. https://doi.org/10.1186/s12913-023-09798-6. Medline:37438778

34 Blauvelt, C., West, M., Maxim, L., Kasiya, A., Dambula, I., Kachila, U., Ngwira, H., & Armstrong, C. E. (2018). Scaling up a health and nutrition hotline in Malawi: The benefits of multisectoral collaboration. *BMJ (Clinical Research Ed.)*, *363*, k4590. https://doi.org/10.1136/bmj.k4590. Medline:30530659

35 Yamey, G., Fewer, S., & Beyeler, N. (2015). Achieving a "grand convergence" in global health by 2035: Rwanda shows the way comment on "Improving the world's health through the post-2015 development agenda: Perspectives from Rwanda." *International Journal of Health Policy and Management*, *4*(11), 789–791. https://doi.org/10.15171/ijhpm.2015.143. Medline:26673345

36 Boyle, C. F., Levin, C., Hatefi, A., Madriz, S., & Santos, N. (2015). Achieving a "grand convergence" in global health: Modeling the technical inputs, costs, and impacts from 2016 to 2030. *PLoS One*, *10*(10), e0140092. https://doi.org/10.1371/journal.pone.0140092. Medline:26452263

37 Simpkin, V., Namubiru-Mwaura, E., Clarke, L., & Mossialos, E. (2019). Investing in health R&D: Where we are, what limits us, and how to make progress in Africa. *BMJ Global Health*, *4*(2), e001047. https://doi.org/10.1136/bmjgh-2018-001047. Medline:30899571

38 Say, L., Chou, D., Gemmill, A., Tunçalp, Ö., Moller, A.-B., Daniels, J., Gülmezoglu, A. M., Temmerman, M., & Alkema, L. (2014). Global causes of maternal death: A WHO systematic analysis. *The Lancet Global Health*, *2*(6), e323–e333. https://doi.org/10.1016/S2214-109X(14)70227-X. Medline:25103301

39 Bartlett, L., Cantor, D., Lynam, P., Kaur, G., Rawlins, B., Ricca, J., Tripathi, V., & Rosen, H. E. (2015). Facility-based active management of the third stage of labour: Assessment of quality in six countries in sub-Saharan Africa. *Bulletin of the World Health Organization, 93*(11), 759–767. https://doi.org/10.2471/BLT.14.142604. Medline:26549903

40 Herrick, T., Mvundura, M., Burke, T. F., & Abu-Haydar, E. (2017). A low-cost uterine balloon tamponade for management of postpartum hemorrhage: Modeling the potential impact on maternal mortality and morbidity in sub-Saharan Africa. *BMC Pregnancy and Childbirth, 17*(1), 374. https://doi.org/10.1186/s12884-017-1564-5. Medline:29132342

41 Jamison, D. T., Summers, L. H., Alleyne, G., Arrow, K. J., Berkley, S., Binagwaho, A., Bustreo, F., Evans, D., Feachem, R. G. A., Frenk, J., Ghosh, G., Goldie, S. J., Guo, Y., Gupta, S., Horton, R., Kruk, M. E., Mahmoud, A., Mohohlo, L. K., Ncube, M., Pablos-Mendez, A., … Yamey, G. (2013). Global health 2035: A world converging within a generation. *The Lancet, 382*(9908), 1898–1955. https://doi.org/10.1016/S0140-6736(13)62105-4. Medline:24309475

42 Kruk, M. E., Yamey, G., Angell, S. Y., Beith, A., Cotlear, D., Guanais, F., Jacobs, L., Saxenian, H., Victora, C., & Goosby, E. (2016). Transforming global health by improving the science of scale-up. *PLoS Biology, 14*(3), e1002360. https://doi.org/10.1371/journal.pbio.1002360. Medline:26934704

43 Whitworth, J., Sewankambo, N. K., & Snewin, V. A. (2010). Improving implementation: Building research capacity in maternal, neonatal, and child health in Africa. *PLoS Medicine, 7*(7), e1000299. https://doi.org/10.1371/journal.pmed.1000299. Medline:20625547

44 Binagwaho, A., & Scott, K. W. (2015). Improving the world's health through the post-2015 development agenda: Perspectives from Rwanda. *International Journal of Health Policy and Management, 4*(4), 203–205. https://doi.org/10.15171/ijhpm.2015.46. Medline:25844381

45 Horwitz, A. (1987). *Comparative public health: Costa Rica, Cuba, and Chile. Food and Nutrition Bulletin, 9*(3). https://archive.unu.edu/unupress/food/8F093e/8F093E04.htm

46 World Bank Group. (2022). *Mortality rate, under-5 (per 1,000 live births).* World Bank Open Data. https://data.worldbank.org

47 Statista. (2021). *R&D: Spending per capita by region 2017.* https://www.statista.com/statistics/1102513/per-capita-research-development-spending-region/

48 Binagwaho, A., Farmer, P. E., Nsanzimana, S., Karema, C., Gasana, M., de Dieu Ngirabega, J., Ngabo, F., Wagner, C. M., Nutt, C. T., Nyatanyi, T., Gatera, M., Kayiteshonga, Y., Mugeni, C., Mugwaneza, P., Shema, J., Uwaliraye, P., Gaju, E., Muhimpundu, M. A., Dushime, T., Senyana, F., … Drobac, P. C. (2014). Rwanda 20 years on: Investing in life. *The Lancet,*

384(9940), 371–375. https://doi.org/10.1016/S0140-6736(14)60574-2. Medline:24703831

49 Msellemu, D., Shemdoe, A., Makungu, C., Mlacha, Y., Kannady, K., Dongus, S., Killeen, G. F., & Dillip, A. (2017). The underlying reasons for very high levels of bed net use, and higher malaria infection prevalence among bed net users than non-users in the Tanzanian city of Dar es Salaam: A qualitative study. *Malaria Journal, 16*(1), 423. https://doi.org/10.1186/s12936-017-2067-6. Medline:29061127

50 Atieli, F. K., Munga, S. O., Ofulla, A. V., & Vulule, J. M. (2010). The effect of repeated washing of long-lasting insecticide-treated nets (LLINs) on the feeding success and survival rates of *Anopheles gambiae.Malaria Journal, 9*(1), 304. https://doi.org/10.1186/1475-2875-9-304. Medline:21029477

51 Lengeler, C. (2004). Insecticide-treated bed nets and curtains for preventing malaria. *Cochrane Database of Systematic Reviews, 2*, CD000363. https://doi.org/10.1002/14651858.CD000363.pub2. Medline:15106149

52 ter Kuile, F. O., Terlouw, D. J., Phillips-Howard, P. A., Hawley, W. A., Friedman, J. F., Kariuki, S. K., Shi, Y. P., Kolczak, M. S., Lal, A. A., Vulule, J. M., & Nahlen, B. L. (2003). Reduction of malaria during pregnancy by permethrin-treated bed nets in an area of intense perennial malaria transmission in western Kenya. *American Journal of Tropical Medicine and Hygiene, 68*(4 Suppl.), 50–60. Medline:12749488

53 UNICEF. (2021). *Malaria in Africa*. https://data.unicef.org/topic/child-health/malaria/

54 Centers for Disease Control and Prevention. (2019, January 28).*How can malaria cases and deaths be reduced? – Insecticide-treated bed nets*.https://www.cdc.gov/malaria/malaria_worldwide/reduction/itn.html.

55 Johansson, E. W., Cibulskis, R. E., Steketee, R. W., & Global Partnership to Roll Back Malaria. (2010). Malaria funding and resource utilization: The first decade of Roll Back Malaria. *Lutte Contre Le Paludisme : Financement et Utilisation Des Ressources : Les Dix Premières Années Du Partenariat RBM Collection Progrès et Impact, 95.*

56 Eisele, T. P., Larsen, D. A., Walker, N., Cibulskis, R. E., Yukich, J. O., Zikusooka, C. M., & Steketee, R. W. (2012). Estimates of child deaths prevented from malaria prevention scale-up in Africa 2001–2010. *Malaria Journal, 11*(1), 93. https://doi.org/10.1186/1475-2875-11-93. Medline:22455864

57 Selemani, M., Msengwa, A. S., Mrema, S., Shamte, A., Mahande, M. J., Yeates, K., Mbago, M. C. Y., & Lutambi, A. M. (2016). Assessing the effects of mosquito nets on malaria mortality using a space time model: A case study of Rufiji and Ifakara Health and Demographic Surveillance System sites in rural Tanzania. *Malaria Journal, 15*(1), 257. https://doi.org/10.1186/s12936-016-1311-9. Medline:27146674

58 Mathieu, E., Ritchie, H., Ortiz-Ospina, E., Roser, M., Hasell, J., Appel, C., Giattino, C., & Rodés-Guirao, L. (2021). A global database of COVID-19 vaccinations. *Nature Human Behaviour*, *5*(7), 947–953. https://doi.org/10.1038/s41562-021-01122-8. Medline:33972767

59 World Health Organization. (2021). *Key lessons from Africa's COVID-19 vaccine rollout. World health Organization. | Regional Office for Africa.* https://www.afro.who.int/news/key-lessons-africas-covid-19-vaccine-rollout

60 Ayenigbara, I. O., Adegboro, J. S., Ayenigbara, G. O., Adeleke, O. R., & Olofintuyi, O. O. (2021). The challenges to a successful COVID-19 vaccination programme in Africa. *Germs*, *11*(3), 427–440. https://doi.org/10.18683/germs.2021.1280. Medline:34722365

61 Jacobson, T. A., Smith, L. E., Hirschhorn, L. R., & Huffman, M. D. (2020). Using implementation science to mitigate worsening health inequities in the United States during the COVID-19 pandemic. *International Journal for Equity in Health*, *19*(1), 170. https://doi.org/10.1186/s12939-020-01293-2. Medline:33004064

62 Ritchie, H., Mathieu, E., Rodés-Guirao, L., Appel, C., Giattino, C., Ortiz-Ospina, E., Hasell, J., Macdonald, B., Beltekian, D., & Roser, M. (2022). *Coronavirus pandemic (COVID-19).* Our World in Data. https://ourworldindata.org/covid-vaccinations

63 Regional Committee for Africa. (2020). *Strategy for scaling up health innovations in the WHO African Region: Report of the Secretariat* (AFR/RC70/11). World Health Organization Regional Office for Africa. https://apps.who.int/iris/handle/10665/333720

64 World Health Organization. (2019). *Winners of inaugural World Health Organization. Innovation Challenge announced.*Regional Office for Africa. https://www.afro.who.int/news/winners-inaugural-who-innovation-challenge-announced

65 African Academy of Sciences. (2022). *Developing excellence in leadership, training and science in Africa (DELTAS Africa).* https://old.aasciences.africa/aesa/programmes/developing-excellence-leadership-training-and-science-africa-deltas-africa

66 Nwaka, S., Ilunga, T. B., Silva, J. S. D., Verde, E. R., Hackley, D., Vré, R. D., Mboya-Okeyo, T., & Ridley, R. G. (2010). Developing ANDI: A novel approach to health product R&D in Africa. *PLOS Medicine*, *7*(6), e1000293. https://doi.org/10.1371/journal.pmed.1000293. Medline:20613865

67 Dutta, S., Lanvin, B., Wunsch-Vincent, S., World Intellectual Property Organization, Insead, Cornell University, & SC Johnson College of Business. (2019). *Global innovation index. Creating healthy lives – The future of medical innovation 2019.*INSEAD. https://www.insead.edu/faculty-research/publications/reports/global-innovation-index-2019-creating-healthy-lives-future

68 World Intellectual Property Organization. (2021). *Global innovation index 2021: Executive summary*. https://www.wipo.int/publications/en/details.jsp?id=4564

69 World Bank. (2021). *Research and development expenditure (% of GDP)*. https://data.worldbank.org/indicator/GB.XPD.RSDV.GD.ZS

70 Diop, O. M. (2017). *Innovation in Africa*. World Bank. https://www.worldbank.org/en/news/speech/2017/11/30/innovation-in-africa

71 Sayagues, M. (2015). Africa's inventors shackled by bad IP regimes. *Appropriate Technology*, *42*(3), 34–35. https://www.scidev.net/global/news/africa-innovation-ip-regimes-aif/

72 New Partnership for Africa's Development. (2003). *Africa's science and technology consolidated plan of action*. Africa Union Common Depository. http://archives.au.int/handle/123456789/5941

73 World Health Organization. (2011). *Implementation research for the control of infectious diseases of poverty: Strengthening the evidence base for the access and delivery of new and improved tools, strategies and interventions*. https://iris.who.int/handle/10665/75216

74 World Health Organization. (2012). *Strategy on health policy and systems research: Changing mindsets*. https://iris.who.int/bitstream/handle/10665/77942/9789241504409_eng.pdf

75 World Health Organization. (2013). *Implementation research in health: A practical guide*. https://iris.who.int/handle/10665/91758

76 Osanjo, G. O., Oyugi, J. O., Kibwage, I. O., Mwanda, W. O., Ngugi, E. N., Otieno, F. C., Ndege, W., Child, M., Farquhar, C., Penner, J., Talib, Z., & Kiarie, J. N. (2016). Building capacity in implementation science research training at the University of Nairobi. *Implementation Science*, *11*(1), 30. https://doi.org/10.1186/s13012-016-0395-5. Medline:26952719

77 Gyamfi, J., Ojo, T., Iwelunmor, J., Ogedegbe, G., Ryan, N., Diawara, A., Nnodu, O., Wonkam, A., Royal, C., & Peprah, E. (2021). Implementation science research for the scale-up of evidence-based interventions for sickle cell disease in Africa: A commentary. *Globalization and Health*, *17*(1), 20. https://doi.org/10.1186/s12992-021-00671-x. Medline:33596947

78 Debaun, M. R., & Galadanci, N. A. (2022, April 4). Sickle cell diseases in Sub-Saharan Africa. *UpToDate*. Retrieved June 26, 2024, from https://www.uptodate.com/contents/sickle-cell-disease-in-sub-saharan-africa

79 Grosse, S. D., Odame, I., Atrash, H. K., Amendah, D. D., Piel, F. B., & Williams, T. N. (2011). Sickle cell disease in Africa: A neglected cause of early childhood mortality. *American Journal of Preventive Medicine*, *41*(6, Suppl. 4), S398–S405. https://doi.org/10.1016/j.amepre.2011.09.013. Medline:22099364

80 Tshilolo, L., Tomlinson, G., Williams, T. N., Santos, B., Olupot-Olupot, P., Lane, A., Aygun, B., Stuber, S. E., Latham, T. S., McGann, P. T., & Ware,

R. E. (2019). Hydroxyurea for children with sickle cell anemia in Sub-Saharan Africa. *New England Journal of Medicine, 380*(2), 121–131. https://doi.org/10.1056/NEJMoa1813598. Medline:30501550

81 Special Programme for Research and Training in Tropical Diseases. (2022). *About us*. https://tdr.who.int/about-us

82 Aurum Institute. (2022). *Implementation research division*. https://www.auruminstitute.org/what-we-do/what-we-do/implementation-research-division

83 Center for Translation and Implementation Research. (2023, October 23). *Research center*. https://ctair.org/

84 Olawepo, J. O., Ezeanolue, E. E., Ekenna, A., Ogunsola, O. O., Itanyi, I. U., Jedy-Agba, E., Egbo, E., Onwuchekwa, C., Ezeonu, A., Ajibola, A., Olakunde, B. O., Majekodunmi, O., Ogidi, A. G., Chukwuorji, J., Lasebikan, N., Dakum, P., Okonkwo, P., Oyeledun, B., Oko, J., … Olutola, A. (2022). Building a national framework for multicentre research and clinical trials: Experience from the Nigeria Implementation Science Alliance. *BMJ Global Health, 7*(4), e008241. https://doi.org/10.1136/bmjgh-2021-008241. Medline:35450861

85 Nigerian Implementation Science Alliance. (n.d.). *Enhancing the quality of health care*. https://nisaresearch.org/

86 Africa Academy for Public Health. (2022). *ARISE network*. https://www.aaph.or.tz/activities/arise-network

87 African Early Childhood Network. (2018). *Implementation research*. https://afecn.org/knowledge-generation

88 Rakhra, A., Mishra, S., Aifah, A., Colvin, C., Gyamfi, J., Ogedegbe, G., & Iwelunmor, J. (2022). Sustaining capacity building and evidence-based NCD intervention implementation: Perspectives from the GRIT consortium. *Frontiers in Health Services*, 2. https://doi.org/10.3389/frhs.2022.891522. Medline:36925894

89 Potter, C., & Brough, R. (2004). Systemic capacity building: A hierarchy of needs. *Health Policy and Planning, 19*(5), 336–345. https://doi.org/10.1093/heapol/czh038

90 Weber, M. B., Baumann, A. A., Rakhra, A., Akwanalo, C., Gladys Amaning Adjei, K., Andesia, J., Apusiga, K., Ha, D. A., Hosseinipour, M. C., Muula, A. S., Nguyen, H. L., Price, L. N., Ramirez-Zea, M., Fitzpatrick, A. L., & Fort, M. P. (2023). Global implementation research capacity building to address cardiovascular disease: An assessment of efforts in eight countries. *PLOS Global Public Health, 3*(9), e0002237. https://doi.org/10.1371/journal.pgph.0002237. Medline:37708090

91 Central and West Africa Implementation Science Alliance. (2022, June 24). *About CAWISA*. https://cawisa-afr.org

92 Water with sugar and salt. (1978). *The Lancet, 312*(8084), 300–301. https://doi.org/10.1016/S0140-6736(78)91698-7

93 World Health Organization. (2006). *Oral rehydration salts production of the new ORS*. https://apps.who.int/iris/bitstream/handle/10665/69227/World health Organization._FCH_CAH_06.1.pdf

94 Binder, H. J., Brown, I., Ramakrishna, B. S., & Young, G. P. (2014). Oral rehydration therapy in the second decade of the twenty-first century. *Current Gastroenterology Reports, 16*(3), 376. https://doi.org/10.1007/s11894-014-0376-2. Medline:24562469

95 Ruxin, J. N. (1994). Magic bullet: The history of oral rehydration therapy. *Medical History, 38*(4), 363–397. https://doi.org/10.1017/S0025727300036905. Medline:7808099

96 Chesney Archives, Johns Hopkins Medicine, Nursing and Public Health. (n.d.). *Daniel C. Darrow collection*. https://medicalarchives.jhmi.edu/collection/daniel-c-darrow-collection/

97 MacIntosh, F. C., & Sourkes, T. L. (1990). Juda Hirsch Quastel. 2 October 1899–15 October 1987. *Biographical Memoirs of Fellows of the Royal Society, 36*, 381–418. Medline:11616176

98 Dadonaite, B. (2019). *Oral rehydration therapy: A low-tech solution that has saved millions of lives*. Our World in Data. https://ourworldindata.org/oral-rehydration-therapy

99 Wolfheim, C., Fontaine, O., & Merson, M. (2019). Evolution of the World Health Organization's programmatic actions to control diarrheal diseases. *Journal of Global Health, 9*(2), 020802. https://doi.org/10.7189/jogh.09.020802. Medline:31673346

100 Hoffman, S. L., Moechtar, M. A., Simanjuntak, C. H., Punjabi, N. H., Kumala, S., Sutoto, Silalahi, P., Sutopo, B., Kuncoro, Y. S., Soriano, M., Plowe, C., Paleologo, F. P., Edman, D. C., & Laughlin, L. W. (1985). Rehydration and maintenance therapy of cholera patients in Jakarta: Citrate-based versus bicarbonate-based oral rehydration salt solution. *Journal of Infectious Diseases, 152*(6), 1159–1165. https://doi.org/10.1093/infdis/152.6.1159. Medline:3905981

101 Islam, M. R. (1986). Citrate can effectively replace bicarbonate in oral rehydration salts for cholera and infantile diarrhoea. *Bulletin of the World Health Organization, 64*(1), 145–150. Medline:3015443

102 World Health Organization. (1999). *The evolution of diarrhoeal and acute respiratory disease control at World Health Organization*. http://apps.who.int/iris/bitstream/handle/10665/66014/World health Organization._CHS_CAH_99.12.pdf

103 World Health Organization. (2004). *Clinical management of acute diarrhoea*. https://apps.who.int/iris/bitstream/handle/10665/68627/World health Organization._FCH_CAH_04.7.pdf

104 World Health Organization. (2009). *Global prevalence of vitamin A deficiency in populations at risk 1995–2005: World Health Organization global database on vitamin A deficiency*. apps.who.int/iris/bitstream/10665/44110/1/9789241598019_eng.pdf

105 Akpede, G. O., Omotara, B. A., Webb, G. D., & Igene, J. O. (1997). Caretakers' knowledge and preparation abilities of salt-sugar solution in north-eastern Nigeria. *Journal of Diarrhoeal Diseases Research, 15*(4), 232–240. Medline:9661319

106 Wiens, K. E., Lindstedt, P. A., Blacker, B. F., Johnson, K. B., Baumann, M. M., Schaeffer, L. E., Abbastabar, H., Abd-Allah, F., Abdelalim, A., Abdollahpour, I., Abegaz, K. H., Abejie, A. N., Abreu, L. G., Abrigo, M. R. M., Abualhasan, A., Accrombessi, M. M. K., Acharya, D., Adabi, M., Adamu, A. A., … Reiner, R. C. (2020). Mapping geographical inequalities in oral rehydration therapy coverage in low-income and middle-income countries, 2000–17. *The Lancet Global Health, 8*(8), e1038–e1060. https://doi.org/10.1016/S2214-109X(20)30230-8. Medline:32710861

107 World Health Organization. (1992). *Programme for control of diarrhoeal diseases: Eighth programme report, 1990–1991*. https://apps.who.int/iris/handle/10665/61647

108 Department of Child and Adolescent Health and Development. (2005). *The treatment of diarrhoea: A manual for physicians and other senior health workers*, 4th ed. World Health Organization. https://iris.who.int/bitstream/handle/10665/43209/9241593180.pdf

109 Centers for Disease Control. (1984). Diarrheal diseases control program: Global activities, 1983. *Morbidity and Mortality Weekly Report, 33*(36), 513–515. Medline:6433166

110 Institute for Health Metrics and Evaluation. (2019). *GBD compare*. http://vizhub.healthdata.org/gbd-compare

111 Boerma, T., Requejo, J., Victora, C. G., Amouzou, A., George, A., Agyepong, I., Barroso, C., Barros, A. J. D., Bhutta, Z. A., Black, R. E., Borghi, J., Buse, K., Aguirre, L. C., Chopra, M., Chou, D., Chu, Y., Claeson, M., Daelmans, B., Davis, A., … Zaidi, S. (2018). Countdown to 2030: Tracking progress towards universal coverage for reproductive, maternal, newborn, and child health. *The Lancet, 391*(10129), 1538–1548. https://doi.org/10.1016/S0140-6736(18)30104-1. Medline:29395268

112 Lenters, L. M., Das, J. K., & Bhutta, Z. A. (2013). Systematic review of strategies to increase use of oral rehydration solution at the household level. *BMC Public Health, 13*(3), S28. https://doi.org/10.1186/1471-2458-13-S3-S28. Medline:24564428

113 Wilson, S. E., Morris, S. S., Gilbert, S. S., Mosites, E., Hackleman, R., Weum, K. L. M., Pintye, J., Manhart, L. E., & Hawes, S. E. (2013). Scaling up access to oral rehydration solution for diarrhea: Learning from

historical experience in low- and high-performing countries. *Journal of Global Health, 3*(1), 010404. https://doi.org/10.7189/jogh.03.010404. Medline:23826508

114 World Health Organization. (2017). Schistosomiasis and soil-transmitted helminthiases: Number of people treated in 2016. *Releve Epidemiologique Hebdomadaire, 92*(49), 749–760. Medline:29218962

115 World Bank. (n.d.). *Diarrhea treatment (% of children under 5 who received ORS packet).* Retrieved October 19, 2024, from https://data.worldbank.org/indicator/SH.STA.ORTH

116 Khan, A. M., Wright, J. E., & Bhutta, Z. A. (2020). A half century of oral rehydration therapy in childhood gastroenteritis: Toward increasing uptake and improving coverage. *Digestive Diseases and Sciences, 65*(2), 355–360. https://doi.org/10.1007/s10620-019-05921-y

117 Ezezika, O., Ragunathan, A., El-Bakri, Y., & Barrett, K. (2021). Barriers and facilitators to implementation of oral rehydration therapy in low- and middle-income countries: A systematic review. *PLOS ONE, 16*(4), e0249638. https://doi.org/10.1371/journal.pone.0249638. Medline:33886584

118 Wilson, S. E., Morris, S. S., & Gilbert, S. S. (2012). *ORS case study Senegal.* Bill and Melinda Gates Foundation. https://healthmarketlinks.org/sites/default/files/resources/Senegal_ORS%20Case%20Study.pdf

119 Derosena, M. (2011). *Challenges in changing diarrhea treatment policy in Senegal* [Technical report].

120 Ellis, A. A., Winch, P., Daou, Z., Gilroy, K. E., & Swedberg, E. (2007). Home management of childhood diarrhoea in southern Mali – Implications for the introduction of zinc treatment. *Social Science & Medicine, 64*(3), 701–712. https://doi.org/10.1016/j.socscimed.2006.10.011. Medline:17097788

121 Gill, S., Hayes, J., & Coates, S. (2012). *From policies to progress: A call for urgent action to prevent the biggest killer of children in sub-Saharan Africa.* Sustainable Sanitation and Water Management Toolbox. https://sswm.info/sites/default/files/reference_attachments/GILL%20et%20al%202012%20DIARRHOEA%20DIALOGUES%20From%20Policies%20to%20Progress.pdf

122 Maxmen, A. (2013). Sierra Leone's free health-care initiative: Work in progress. *Lancet (London, England), 381*(9862), 191–192. https://doi.org/10.1016/s0140-6736(13)60074-4. Medline:23346591

123 Diaz, T., George, A. S., Rao, S. R., Bangura, P. S., Baimba, J. B., McMahon, S. A., & Kabano, A. (2013). Healthcare seeking for diarrhoea, malaria and pneumonia among children in four poor rural districts in Sierra Leone in the context of free health care: Results of a cross-sectional survey. *BMC Public Health, 13*(1), 157. https://doi.org/10.1186/1471-2458-13-157. Medline:23425576

124 Prins, A. (1989). *Review of the Malawi CDD program*. USAID. https://pdf.usaid.gov/pdf_docs/PNABM300.pdf

125 Danart, A., Mackie, W., Cisek, C., Kondoole, N., & Chizani, N. (2004). *Population Services International's improving health through social marketing project executive summary*. USAID. https://pdf.usaid.gov/pdf_docs/Pdacd081.pdf

126 Federal Republic of Nigeria. (2012). *Essential childhood medicines scale-up plan, 2012–2015*. Federal Ministry of Health, & National Primary Health Care Development Agency. https://www.childhealthtaskforce.org/sites/default/files/2019-05/Essential%20Childhood%20Medicines%20Scale-Up%20Plan%28Federal%20Ministry%20of%20Health%2CNational%20Primary%20Health%20Care%20Development%20Agency%2C%202012%29.pdf

127 Clinton Health Access Initiative. (2017). *Shaping local markets to scale-up zinc and ORS in Nigeria*. https://clintonhealthaccess.org/wp-content/uploads/2017/07/2137-EM-Program-Overview-with-State-Briefs-v9TC-SCREEN_FINAL.pdf

128 Miller, P., & Hirschhorn, N. (1995). The effect of a national control of diarrheal diseases program on mortality: The case of Egypt. *Social Science & Medicine (1982)*, *40*(10), S1–S30. https://doi.org/10.1016/0277-9536(95)00001-n. Medline:7638641

129 GiveWell. (2009). *Case study: Oral rehydration solution (ORS)*. https://files.givewell.org/files/DWDA%202009/Interventions/ORS/MS_case_8.pdf

130 Levine, R. (n.d.). *Case 8: Preventing Diarrheal Deaths in Egypt*. https://files.givewell.org/files/DWDA%202009/Interventions/ORS/MS_case_8.pdf

131 Lam, F., Abdulwahab, A., Houdek, J., Adekeye, O., Abubakar, M., Akinjeji, A., Braimoh, T., Ajeroh, O., Stanley, M., Goh, N., Schroder, K., Wiwa, O., Ihebuzor, N., & Prescott, M. R. (2019). Program evaluation of an ORS and zinc scale-up program in 8 Nigerian states. *Journal of Global Health*, *9*(1), 010502. https://doi.org/10.7189/jogh.09.010502. Medline:31073399

132 Wagner, Z., Asiimwe, J. B., Dow, W. H., & Levine, D. I. (2019). The role of price and convenience in use of oral rehydration salts to treat child diarrhea: A cluster randomized trial in Uganda. *PLoS Medicine*, *16*(1), e1002734. https://doi.org/10.1371/journal.pmed.1002734

133 Donnelly, J. (2011). How did Sierra Leone provide free health care? *The Lancet*, *377*(9775), 1393–1396. https://doi.org/10.1016/S0140-6736(11)60559-X. Medline:21520507

134 Kassegne, S., Kays, M. B., & Nzohabonayo, J. (2011). Evaluation of a social marketing intervention promoting oral rehydration salts in Burundi. *BMC Public Health*, *11*(1), 155. https://doi.org/10.1186/1471-2458-11-155. Medline:21385460

135 Morris, S., Gilbert, S., & Wilson, S. (2012). *ORS case study Malawi.* https://healthmarketlinks.org/sites/default/files/resources/Malawi_ORS%20Case%20Study.pdf
136 Munthali, A. C. (2005). Change and continuity in the management of diarrhoeal diseases in under-five children in rural Malawi. *Malawi Medical Journal, 16*(2), 43–46. https://doi.org/10.4314/mmj.v16i2.10859
137 National Statistical Office & ICF Macro. (2011). *Malawi Demographic and Health Survey 2010.* https://dhsprogram.com/pubs/pdf/FR247/FR247.pdf
138 Kenya, P. R., Gatiti, S., Muthami, L. N., Agwanda, R., Mwenesi, H. A., Katsivo, M. N., Omondi-Odhiambo, null, Surrow, A., Juma, R., & Ellison, R. H. (1990). Oral rehydration therapy and social marketing in rural Kenya. *Social Science & Medicine (1982), 31*(9), 979–987. https://doi.org/10.1016/0277-9536(90)90107-4. Medline:2255970
139 Charyeva, Z., Cannon, M., Oguntunde, O., Garba, A. M., Sambisa, W., Bassi, A. P., Ibrahim, M. A., Danladi, S. E., & Lawal, N. (2015). Reducing the burden of diarrhea among children under five years old: Lessons learned from oral rehydration therapy corner program implementation in Northern Nigeria. *Journal of Health, Population and Nutrition, 34*(1), 4. https://doi.org/10.1186/s41043-015-0005-1. Medline:26825053
140 Elias, C. J. (2016). *Solutions to defeat a global killer.* PATH. http://www.path.org/publications/files/IMM_solutions_global_killer.pdf
141 Kassegne, S., & Nzohabonayo, J. (2011). *Burundi (2007): TRaC study to evaluate the use of Orasel in women with children under 5 years of age. Second round.* Harvard Dataverse, V4. https://doi.org/10.7910/DVN/TAEEZ8
142 Dippenaar, H., Joubert, G., Nel, R., Bantobetse, M., Opawole, A., & Roshen, K. (2005). Homemade sugar-salt solution for oral rehydration: Knowledge of mothers and caregivers. *South African Family Practice, 47*(2), 51–53. https://doi.org/10.1080/20786204.2005.10873188
143 SHOPS Project. (2015). *Ghana program profile.* Abt Associates. https://pdf.usaid.gov/pdf_docs/PA00KZVV.pdf
144 Gebremedhin, S., Mamo, G., Gezahign, H., Kung'u, J., & Adish, A. (2016). The effectiveness bundling of zinc with Oral Rehydration Salts (ORS) for improving adherence to acute watery diarrhea treatment in Ethiopia: Cluster randomised controlled trial. *BMC Public Health, 16*(1), 457. https://doi.org/10.1186/s12889-016-3126-6. Medline:27246705
145 Kassaye, M., Larson, C., & Carlson, D. (1994). A randomized community trial of prepackaged and homemade oral rehydration therapies. *Archives of Pediatrics & Adolescent Medicine, 148*(12), 1288–1292. https://doi.org/10.1001/archpedi.1994.02170120050008. Medline:7951808
146 Teferedegn, B., Larson, C. P., & Carlson, D. (1993). A community-based randomized trial of homemade oral rehydration therapies. *International*

Journal of Epidemiology, 22(5), 917–922. https://doi.org/10.1093/ije/22.5.917. Medline:8282473

147 Brauer, M., Zhao, J. T., Bennitt, F. B., & Stanaway, J. D. (2020). Global access to handwashing: Implications for COVID-19 control in low-income countries. *Environmental Health Perspectives, 128*(5), 057005. https://doi.org/10.1289/EHP7200. Medline:32438824

148 Kisaakye, P., Ndagurwa, P., & Mushomi, J. (2021). An assessment of the availability of handwashing facilities in households from four East African countries. *Journal of Water, Sanitation and Hygiene for Development, 11*(1), 75–90. https://doi.org/10.2166/washdev.2020.129

149 Jiwani, S. S., & Antiporta, D. A. (2020). Inequalities in access to water and soap matter for the COVID-19 response in sub-Saharan Africa. *International Journal for Equity in Health, 19*(1), 82. https://doi.org/10.1186/s12939-020-01199-z. Medline:32493409

150 Freeman, M. C., Stocks, M. E., Cumming, O., Jeandron, A., Higgins, J. P., Wolf, J., Prüss-Ustün, A., Bonjour, S., Hunter, P. R., Fewtrell, L., & Curtis, V. (2014). Systematic review: Hygiene and health: Systematic review of handwashing practices worldwide and update of health effects. *Tropical Medicine & International Health, 19*(8), 906–916.

151 Martini, M., & Lippi, D. (2021). SARS-CoV-2 (COVID-19) and the teaching of Ignaz Semmelweis and Florence Nightingale: A lesson of public health from history, after the "introduction of handwashing" (1847). *Journal of Preventive Medicine and Hygiene, 62*(3), E621. https://doi.org/10.15167/2421-4248/jpmh2021.62.3.2161. Medline:34909488

152 Newsom, S. W. B. (2001). The history of infection control: Semmelweis and handwashing. *British Journal of Infection Control,* 2(4), 24–25.

153 Ataman, A. D., Vatanoğlu-Lutz, E. E., & Yıldırım, G. (2013). Medicine in stamps-Ignaz Semmelweis and puerperal fever. *Journal of the Turkish German Gynecological Association, 14*(1), 35. https://doi.org/10.5152/jtgga.2013.08. Medline:24592068

154 National Research Council (US) Committee to Update Science, Medicine, and Animals. (2004). *Science, medicine, and animals.* National Academies Press. http://www.ncbi.nlm.nih.gov/books/NBK24656/

155 Duka, T. (1886). Childbed fever, its causes and prevention: A life's history. *The Lancet, 128*(3283), 206–208. https://doi.org/10.1016/S0140-6736(00)49790-4

156 Nightingale, F. (1860). *Notes on nursing: What it is, and what it is not.* D, Appleton and Company. https://digital.library.upenn.edu/women/nightingale/nursing/nursing.html

157 Larson, E. L., Quiros, D., & Lin, S. X. (2007). Dissemination of the CDC's Hand Hygiene Guideline and impact on infection rates. *American Journal*

of Infection Control, *35*(10), 666–675. https://doi.org/10.1016/j.ajic.2006.10.006. Medline:18063132

158 Garner, J. S., & Favero, M. S. (1985). *Guideline for handwashing and hospital environmental control, 1985*. https://www.ospedalesicuro.eu/storia/materiali/doc/Handwashing.html

159 Haas, J. P., & Larson, E. L. (2008). Compliance with hand hygiene guidelines: Where are we in 2008? *American Journal of Nursing*, *108*(8), 40–44. https://doi.org/10.1097/01.NAJ.0000330260.76229.71. Medline:18664758

160 World Health Organization. (2009). *Guidelines on hand hygiene in health care*. https://iris.who.int/bitstream/handle/10665/44102/9789241597906_eng.pdf

161 World Health Organization. (2021). *World hand hygiene day*. https://www.who.int/campaigns/world-hand-hygiene-day

162 World Health Organization. (2018). *Millennium Development Goals (MDGs)*. https://www.who.int/news-room/fact-sheets/detail/millennium-development-goals-(mdgs)

163 Gunnlaugsson, G., Einarsdóttir, J., Angulo, F. J., Mentambanar, S. A., Passa, A., & Tauxe, R. V. (1998). Funerals during the 1994 cholera epidemic in Guinea-Bissau, West Africa: The need for disinfection of bodies of persons dying of cholera. *Epidemiology & Infection*, *120*(1), 7–15. https://doi.org/10.1017/s0950268897008170. Medline:9528812

164 Mulholland, K. (1985). Cholera in Sudan: An account of an epidemic in a refugee camp in eastern Sudan, May–June 1985. *Disasters*, *9*(4), 247–258. https://doi.org/10.1111/j.1467-7717.1985.tb00947.x. Medline:20958607

165 Cobra, C., & Sack, D. A. (1996). *The control of epidemic dysentery in Africa: Overview, recommendations, and checklists*. US Agency for International Development, Bureau for Africa, Office of Sustainable Development, Human Resources and Democracy Division.

166 United Nations. (n.d.). *Water and sanitation*. https://sdgs.un.org/topics/water-and-sanitation

167 Global Handwashing Partnership. (n.d.). *Who we are*. https://globalhandwashing.org/about-us/who-we-are/

168 Alzyood, M., Jackson, D., Aveyard, H., & Brooke, J. (2020). COVID-19 reinforces the importance of handwashing. *Journal of Clinical Nursing*, *29*(15–16), 2760. https://doi.org/10.1111/jocn.15313. Medline:32406958

169 Erasmus, V., Daha, T. J., Brug, H., Richardus, J. H., Behrendt, M. D., Vos, M. C., & van Beeck, E. F. (2010). A systematic review of studies on compliance with hand hygiene guidelines in hospital care. *Infection Control & Hospital Epidemiology*, *31*(3), 283–294. https://doi.org/10.1086/650451. Medline:20088678

170 Global Handwashing Partnership. (n.d.). *What we do*. https://globalhandwashing.org/about-us/what-we-do/

171 World Health Organization. (2020). *Hand hygiene for all global initiative*. https://www.who.int/initiatives/hand-hygiene-for-all-global-initiative

172 World Bank. (2020). *COVID-19 makes handwashing facilities and promotion more critical than ever*. https://www.worldbank.org/en/news/feature/2020/04/30/covid-19-makes-handwashing-facilities-and-promotion-more-critical-than-ever

173 World Bank. (2019). *Indonesia: Expanding access to clean water for the rural poor*. https://www.worldbank.org/en/results/2019/07/29/indonesia-expanding-access-to-clean-water-for-the-rural-poor

174 Ndegwa, L., Hatfield, K. M., Sinkowitz-Cochran, R., D'Iorio, E., Gupta, N., Kimotho, J., Woodard, T., Chaves, S. S., & Ellingson, K. (2019). Evaluation of a program to improve hand hygiene in Kenyan hospitals through production and promotion of alcohol-based handrub – 2012–2014. *Antimicrobial Resistance & Infection Control*, *8*, 1–6. https://doi.org/10.1186/s13756-018-0450-x. Medline:30622703

175 World Health Organization. (2020). *Guidance for climate resilient and environmentally sustainable health care facilities*. https://apps.who.int/iris/handle/10665/335909

176 Infection Control Africa Network. (n.d.). *Turn Africa Orange initiative*. Retrieved April 15, 2024 from: https://icanetwork.co.za/turn-africa-orange-initiative/

177 Centers for Disease Control and Prevention. (n.d.). *Mobile handwashing stations launched to fight COVID-19*. https://archive.cdc.gov/#/details?q=https://www.cdc.gov/globalhealth/stories/2020/covid-mobile-handwashing-stations.html&start=0&rows=10&url=https://www.cdc.gov/globalhealth/stories/2020/covid-mobile-handwashing-stations.html

178 US Mission South Africa. (2020). *US PEPFAR funds local handwashing innovation Shesha Geza*. U.S. Embassy & Consulates in South Africa. https://za.usembassy.gov/u-s-pepfar-funds-local-handwashing-innovation-shesha-geza/

179 Aurum Innova. (n.d.). *About us*. https://www.auruminnova.com/about-us/

180 UNICEF. (2020). *UNICEF launches "Tippy Tap" challenge to mobilise young people against surging COVID-19 cases*. https://www.unicef.org/southafrica/press-releases/unicef-launches-tippy-tap-challenge-mobilise-young-people-against-surging-covid-19

181 WaterAid. (2018). *State of hygiene in Southern Africa: Summary of Key findings*. https://washmatters.wateraid.org/sites/g/files/jkxoof256/files/State%20of%20Hygiene%20in%20South%20Africa.pdf

182 Greater Accra Metropolitan Area Sanitation & Water Project. (n.d.). *Greater Accra Metropolitan Area sanitation and water project (GAMA-SWP).* https://www.gamaswp.org/about-us/
183 Kar, K., & Chambers, R. (2008). *Handbook on community-led total sanitation (CLTS).* Plan International. https://plan-international.org/uploads/2022/01/2008_handbook_on_community_led_total_sanitation_en.pdf
184 Venkataramanan, V., Crocker, J., Karon, A., & Bartram, J. (2018). Community-led total sanitation: A mixed-methods systematic review of evidence and its quality. *Environmental Health Perspectives, 126*(2), 026001. https://doi.org/10.1289/EHP1965. Medline:29398655
185 Crocker, J., Saywell, D., & Bartram, J. (2017). Sustainability of community-led total sanitation outcomes: Evidence from Ethiopia and Ghana. *International Journal of Hygiene and Environmental Health, 220*(3), 551–557. https://doi.org/10.1016/j.ijheh.2017.02.011. Medline:28522255
186 Muchangi, M., & Kimathi, G. (2017). Lessons learnt from implementation of outcome linked community led total sanitation intervention in Busia Kenya. In R. J. Shaw (Ed.), *Local action with international cooperation to improve and sustain water, sanitation and hygiene (WASH) services: Proceedings of the 40th WEDC international conference.* CORE: Loughborough University Institutional Repository. https://core.ac.uk/download/pdf/288362725.pdf
187 Mbakaya, B. C., Kalembo, F. W., & Zgambo, M. (2020). Use, adoption, and effectiveness of tippy-tap handwashing station in promoting hand hygiene practices in resource-limited settings: A systematic review. *BMC Public Health, 20*(1), 1005. https://doi.org/10.1186/s12889-020-09101-w. Medline:32586314
188 Biran, A. (2011). *Enabling technologies for handwashing with soap: a case study on the tippy-tap in Uganda.* Global Handwashing Partnership. https://globalhandwashing.org/wp-content/uploads/2015/03/uganda-tippy-tap-hwws.pdf
189 Zhang, C., Mosa, A. J., Hayward, A. S., & Matthews, S. A. (2013). Promoting clean hands among children in Uganda: A school-based intervention using "tippy-taps." *Public Health, 127*(6), 586. https://doi.org/10.1016/j.puhe.2012.10.020. Medline:23267769
190 One Drop Foundation. (n.d.). *Everything about our unique social art for behaviour change approach.* https://www.onedrop.org/en/everything-about-our-unique-social-art-for-behaviour-change-approach/
191 WaterAid. (2018). *WaterAid Mali annual report.* https://www.wateraid.org/ca/sites/g/files/jkxoof281/files/2018-08/18282_wateraid_mali_annual_report_2017_18_EN_PRINT.pdf

192 One Drop Foundation. (n.d.). *Results*. https://www.onedrop.org/en/results/

193 World Water Week. (n.d.). *Social art for behaviour change: Contributing towards achievement of SDG6*. https://www.worldwaterweek.org/event/8629-social-art-for-behaviour-change-contributing-towards-achievement-of-sdg6

194 Sultana, F., Unicomb, L. E., Nizame, F. A., Dutta, N. C., Ram, P. K., Luby, S. P., & Winch, P. J. (2018). Acceptability and feasibility of sharing a soapy water system for Handwashing in a low-income urban community in Dhaka, Bangladesh: A qualitative study. *American Journal of Tropical Medicine and Hygiene*, *99*(2), 502. https://doi.org/10.4269/ajtmh.17-0672. Medline:29893204

195 Innovations for Poverty Action. (2017). *Soapy water handwashing stations final report*. https://pdf.usaid.gov/pdf_docs/pa00srv2.pdf

196 Ezezika, O., Heng, J., Fatima, K., Mohamed, A., & Barrett, K. (2023). What are the barriers and facilitators to community handwashing with water and soap? A systematic review. *PLOS Global Public Health*, *3*(4), e0001720. https://doi.org/10.1371/journal.pgph.0001720. Medline:37074999

197 Lankford, M. G., Zembower, T. R., Trick, W. E., Hacek, D. M., Noskin, G. A., & Peterson, L. R. (2003). Influence of role models and hospital design on the hand hygiene of health-care workers. *Emerging Infectious Diseases*, *9*(2), 217. https://doi.org/10.3201/eid0902.020249. Medline:12603993

198 Sands, M., & Aunger, R. (2020). *Determinants of Hand Hygiene Compliance Among Nurses in US Hospitals: A Formative Research Study. PLoS One*, *15*(4), Article e0230573. https://doi.org/10.1371/journal.pone.0230573. Medline:32255783

199 Hartford, D. (n.d.). *Thousands of youth take up the #TippyTapChallenge: A handwashing solution making a targeted splash in South Africa*. UNICEF South Africa. https://www.unicef.org/southafrica/stories/thousands-youth-take-tippytapchallenge

200 Naughton, C. C., Sissoko, H. T., & Mihelcic, J. R. (2015). Assessing factors that lead to use of appropriate technology handwashing stations in Mali, West Africa. *Journal of Water, Sanitation and Hygiene for Development*, *5*(2), 279–288. https://doi.org/10.2166/washdev.2015.135

201 Biran, A., Schmidt, W. P., Zeleke, L., Emukule, H., Khay, H., Parker, J., & Peprah, D. (2012). Hygiene and sanitation practices amongst residents of three long-term refugee camps in Thailand, Ethiopia and Kenya. *Tropical Medicine & International Health*, *17*(9), 1133–1141. https://doi.org/10.1111/j.1365-3156.2012.03045.x. Medline:22845619

202 Amunga, V. (2021). *To encourage handwashing, Kenyan charity makes vegetable soap for the poor*. VOA News. https://www.voanews.com/a/covid-19-pandemic_encourage-handwashing-kenyan-charity-makes-vegetable-soap-poor/6204324.html

203 Rabin, B. A., & Brownson, R. C. (2017). Terminology for dissemination and implementation research. *Dissemination and Implementation Research in Health: Translating Science to Practice*, 2, 19–45. https://doi.org/10.1093/oso/9780190683214.003.0002

204 Holmen, I. C., Niyokwizerwa, D., Nyiranzayisaba, B., Singer, T., & Safdar, N. (2017). Challenges to sustainability of hand hygiene at a rural hospital in Rwanda. *American Journal of Infection Control*, *45*(8), 855–859. https://doi.org/10.1016/j.ajic.2017.04.006. Medline:28596020

205 Wichaidit, W., Steinacher, R., Okal, J. A., Whinnery, J., Null, C., Kordas, K., Yu, J., Pickering, A. J., & Ram, P. K. (2019). Effect of an equipment-behavior change intervention on handwashing behavior among primary school children in Kenya: The Povu Poa school pilot study. *BMC Public Health*, *19*, 1–12. https://doi.org/10.1186/s12889-019-6902-2. Medline:31138168

206 Alexander, K. T., Dreibelbis, R., Freeman, M. C., Ojeny, B., & Rheingans, R. (2013). Improving service delivery of water, sanitation, and hygiene in primary schools: A cluster-randomized trial in western Kenya. *Journal of Water and Health*, *11*(3), 507–519. https://doi.org/10.2166/wh.2013.213. Medline:23981878

207 Saboori, S., Greene, L. E., Moe, C. L., Freeman, M. C., Caruso, B. A., Akoko, D., & Rheingans, R. D. (2013). Impact of regular soap provision to primary schools on hand washing and E. coli hand contamination among pupils in Nyanza Province, Kenya: A cluster-randomized trial. *American Journal of Tropical Medicine and Hygiene*, *89*(4), 698. https://doi.org/10.4269/ajtmh.12-0387. Medline:23939707

208 Chittleborough, C. R., Nicholson, A. L., Basker, E., Bell, S., & Campbell, R. (2012). Factors influencing hand washing behaviour in primary schools: Process evaluation within a randomized controlled trial. *Health Education Research*, *27*(6), 1055–1068. https://doi.org/10.1093/her/cys061. Medline:22623617

209 La Con, G., Schilling, K., Harris, J., Person, B., Owuor, M., Ogange, L., Faith, S., & Quick, R. (2017). Evaluation of student handwashing practices during a school-based hygiene program in rural Western Kenya, 2007. *International Quarterly of Community Health Education*, *37*(2), 121–128. https://doi.org/10.1177/0272684X17701263. Medline:28511602

210 World Vision. (2020). *Merlin gets serious on hand washing; confides, "Mothers in Juba are terrified of coronavirus."* https://www.wvi.org/stories/coronavirus-health-crisis/merlin-gets-serious-hand-washing-confides-mothers-juba-are

211 Okello, E., Kapiga, S., Grosskurth, H., Makata, K., Mcharo, O., Kinungh'i, S., & Dreibelbis, R. (2019). Factors perceived to facilitate or hinder handwashing among primary students: A qualitative assessment

of the Mikono Safi intervention schools in NW Tanzania. *BMJ Open*, *9*(11), e030947. https://doi.org/10.1136/bmjopen-2019-030947. Medline:31784435

212 Hotez, P. J. (2012). *Inspiring a generation of women to fight neglected tropical diseases*. HuffPost. https://www.huffpost.com/entry/maternal-health-ntds_b_1318335.

213 Andrews, P., Thomas, H., Pohlke, R., & Seubert, Jür. (1983). Praziquantel. *Medicinal Research Reviews*, *3*(2), 147–200. https://doi.org/10.1002/med.2610030204. Medline:6408323

214 Groll, E. (1984). Praziquantel. *Advances in Pharmacology and Chemotherapy*, *20*, 219–238. https://doi.org/10.1016/s1054-3589(08)60268-9. Medline:6398968

215 Reich, M. R., & Govindaraj, R. (1998). Dilemmas in drug development for tropical diseases: Experiences with praziquantel. *Health Policy*, *44*(1), 1–18. https://doi.org/10.1016/s0168-8510(98)00002-5. Medline:10180198

216 King, C. H., & Mahmoud, A. A. F. (1989). Drugs five years later: Praziquantel. *Annals of Internal Medicine*, *110*(4), 290–296. https://doi.org/10.7326/0003-4819-110-4-290. Medline:2643915

217 Liu, L. X., & Weller, P. F. (1996). Antiparasitic drugs. *New England Journal of Medicine*, *334*(18), 1178–1184. https://doi.org/10.1056/NEJM199605023341808

218 World Health Organization. (1984). *The control of schistosomiasis: Report of World Health Organization expert committee*. Technical Report Series No. 728. https://www.who.int/publications/i/item/WHO-TRS-728

219 el Malatawy, A., el Habashy, A., Lechine, N., Dixon, H., Davis, A., & Mott, K. E. (1992). Selective population chemotherapy among schoolchildren in Beheira governorate: The UNICEF/Arab Republic of Egypt/WHO Schistosomiasis Control Project. *Bulletin of the World Health Organization*, *70*(1), 47–56. Medline:1568280

220 Farag, M. K., el-Shazly, A. M., Khashaba, M. T., & Attia, R. A. (1993). Impact of the current National Bilharzia Control Programme on the epidemiology of schistosomiasis mansoni in an Egyptian village. *Transactions of the Royal Society of Tropical Medicine and Hygiene*, *87*(3), 250–253. https://doi.org/10.1016/0035-9203(93)90112-4. Medline:8236381

221 Stothard, J. R., Sousa-Figueiredo, J. C., Betson, M., Green, H. K., Seto, E. Y. W., Garba, A., Sacko, M., Mutapi, F., Vaz Nery, S., Amin, M. A., Mutumba-Nakalembe, M., Navaratnam, A., Fenwick, A., Kabatereine, N. B., Gabrielli, A. F., & Montresor, A. (2011). Closing the praziquantel treatment gap: New steps in epidemiological monitoring and control of schistosomiasis in African infants and preschool-aged children. *Parasitology*, *138*(12), 1593–1606. https://doi.org/10.1017/S0031182011001235. Medline:21861945

222 Tchuem Tchuenté, L.-A., Rollinson, D., Stothard, J. R., & Molyneux, D. (2017). Moving from control to elimination of schistosomiasis in sub-Saharan Africa: Time to change and adapt strategies. *Infectious Diseases of Poverty*, *6*(1), 42. https://doi.org/10.1186/s40249-017-0256-8. Medline:28219412

223 Kokaliaris, C., Garba, A., Matuska, M., Bronzan, R. N., Colley, D. G., Dorkenoo, A. M., Ekpo, U. F., Fleming, F. M., French, M. D., Kabore, A., Mbonigaba, J. B., Midzi, N., Mwinzi, P. N. M., N'Goran, E. K., Polo, M. R., Sacko, M., Tchuenté, L.-A. T., Tukahebwa, E. M., Uvon, P. A., … Vounatsou, P. (2022). Effect of preventive chemotherapy with Praziquantel on schistosomiasis among school-aged children in sub-Saharan Africa: A spatiotemporal modelling study. *The Lancet Infectious Diseases*, *22*(1), 136–149. https://doi.org/10.1016/S1473-3099(21)00090-6. Medline:34863336

224 World Health Organization. (2021). *Ending the neglect to attain the Sustainable Development Goals: A road map for neglected tropical diseases 2021–2030*. https://www.who.int/publications/i/item/9789240010352

225 Obonyo, C. O., Muok, E. M., & Were, V. (2019). Biannual praziquantel treatment for schistosomiasis. *Cochrane Database of Systematic Reviews*, *2019*(8), CD013412. https://doi.org/10.1002/14651858.CD013412

226 Doenhoff, M. J., Hagan, P., Cioli, D., Southgate, V., Pica-Mattoccia, L., Botros, S., Coles, G., Tchuem Tchuenté, L. A., Mbaye, A., & Engels, D. (2009). Praziquantel: Its use in control of schistosomiasis in sub-Saharan Africa and current research needs. *Parasitology*, *136*(13), 1825–1835. https://doi.org/10.1017/S0031182009000493. Medline:19281637

227 World Health Organization. (2019). Schistosomiasis and soil-transmitted helminthiases: Numbers of people treated in 2018. *Weekly Epidemiological Record*, *94*, 601–612. https://www.who.int/publications/i/item/who-wer9450

228 World Health Organization. (2022). *World Health Organization guideline on control and elimination of human schistosomiasis*. https://www.who.int/publications-detail-redirect/9789240041608

229 World Health Organization. (2016). Summary of global update on preventive chemotherapy implementation in 2015. *Weekly Epidemiological Record*, *91*(39), 456–460. Medline:27758092

230 World Health Organization. (2001). *World Health Assembly endorses World Health Organization's strategic priorities*. https://www.who.int/news/item/22-05-2001-world-health-assembly-endorses-who-s-strategic-priorities

231 World Health Organization. (2013). *Schistosomiasis: Progress report 2001–2011 and strategic plan 2012–2020*. https://apps.who.int/iris/handle/10665/78074

232 Rebollo, M. P., Onyeze, A. N., Tiendrebeogo, A., Senkwe, M. N., Impouma, B., Ogoussan, K., Zouré, H. G. M., Deribe, K., Cano, J., Kinvi, E. B., Majewski, A., Ottesen, E. A., & Lammie, P. (2021). Baseline mapping of neglected tropical diseases in Africa: The accelerated WHO/AFRO mapping project. *American Journal of Tropical Medicine and Hygiene, 104*(6), 2298–2304. https://doi.org/10.4269/ajtmh.20-1538. Medline:33901001

233 Garba, A., Touré, S., Dembelé, R., Bosque-Oliva, E., & Fenwick, A. (2006). Implementation of national schistosomiasis control programmes in West Africa. *Trends in Parasitology, 22*(7), 322–326. https://doi.org/10.1016/j.pt.2006.04.007. Medline:16690357

234 World Health Organization. (2021). *PCT Databank – schistosomiasis*. https://www.who.int/teams/control-of-neglected-tropical-diseases/data-platforms/pct-databank/schistosomiasis

235 Hotez, P. J., & Kamath, A. (2009). Neglected tropical diseases in sub-Saharan Africa: Review of their prevalence, distribution, and disease burden. *PLoS Neglected Tropical Diseases, 3*(8), e412. https://doi.org/10.1371/journal.pntd.0000412. Medline:19707588

236 Hotez, P. J., Engels, D., Fenwick, A., & Savioli, L. (2010). Africa is desperate for Praziquantel. *Lancet (London, England), 376*(9740), 496–498. https://doi.org/10.1016/S0140-6736(10)60879-3. Medline:20709217

237 Fenwick, A., Webster, J. P., Bosque-Oliva, E., Blair, L., Fleming, F. M., Zhang, Y., Garba, A., Stothard, J. R., Gabrielli, A. F., Clements, A. C. A., Kabatereine, N. B., Toure, S., Dembele, R., Nyandindi, U., Mwansa, J., & Koukounari, A. (2009). The Schistosomiasis Control Initiative (SCI): Rationale, development and implementation from 2002–2008. *Parasitology, 136*(13), 1719–1730. https://doi.org/10.1017/S0031182009990400. Medline:19631008

238 Merck KGaA. (2022, January 24). *Merck KGaA, Darmstadt, Germany, provides 1.5 billionth tablet of praziquantel for treatment of schistosomiasis* [Press release]. https://www.merckgroup.com/en/news/praziquantel-tablet-donation-24-01-2022.html

239 Kabatereine, N. B., Fleming, F. M., Nyandindi, U., Mwanza, J. C. L., & Blair, L. (2006). The control of schistosomiasis and soil-transmitted helminths in East Africa. *Trends in Parasitology, 22*(7), 332–339. https://doi.org/10.1016/j.pt.2006.05.001. Medline:16713357

240 Carter Center. (n.d.). *Schistosomiasis (bilharziasis)control program*. https://www.cartercenter.org/health/schistosomiasis/index.html

241 CBM Neglected Tropical Diseases (2020). *Annual report: Ensuring access for all.* 2020. https://www.cbm.org/fileadmin/user_upload/CBM_NTD_Report_2018_FINAL.pdf

242 SightSavers. (2020). *Sightsavers deworming program—Nigeria, Yobe State GiveWell wishlist 4 schistosomiasis (SCH)/soil transmitted helminth (STH)*

project narrative. https://files.givewell.org/files/DWDA%202009/Sightsavers/Sightsavers_Nigeria_Yobe_State_Wishlist_4_country_narrative_2019.pdf

243 United Nations (2012, November 8). *Three million Nigerians to benefit from life-saving de-worming tablets donated by the UN* [News release]. https://news.un.org/en/story/2012/11/425072-three-million-nigerians-benefit-life-saving-de-worming-tablets-donated-un

244 Ezezika, O., Nebe, O. J., Gong, J., Surakat, O., Ogoji, J. O., & Aladesanmi, O. (2024). Implementation of school-based mass drug administration of praziquantel in Nigeria: Barriers, facilitators, and opportunities for improvement [Manuscript submitted for publication].

245 Mazigo, H. D., Nuwaha, F., Kinung'hi, S. M., Morona, D., de Moira, A. P., Wilson, S., Heukelbach, J., & Dunne, D. W. (2012). Epidemiology and control of human schistosomiasis in Tanzania. *Parasites & Vectors*, *5*(1), 274. https://doi.org/10.1186/1756-3305-5-274. Medline:23192005

246 Savioli, L., Dixon, H., Kisumku, U. M., & Mott, K. E. (1989). Control of morbidity due to Schistosoma haematobium on Pemba Island: Programme organization and management. *Tropical Medicine and Parasitology: Official Organ of Deutsche Tropenmedizinische Gesellschaft and of Deutsche Gesellschaft Fur Technische Zusammenarbeit (GTZ)*, *40*(2), 189–194. Medline:2505381

247 Ministry of Health and Social Welfare Tanzania Mainland. (2010). *Report on urinary schistosomiasis, national questionnaire baseline survey in Tanzania mainland 2010*. Schistosomiasis Control Initiatives.

248 Damschroder, L. J., Aron, D. C., Keith, R. E., Kirsh, S. R., Alexander, J. A., & Lowery, J. C. (2009). Fostering implementation of health services research findings into practice: A consolidated framework for advancing implementation science. *Implementation Science: IS*, *4*, 50. https://doi.org/10.1186/1748-5908-4-50. Medline:19664226

249 Keith, R. E., Crosson, J. C., O'Malley, A. S., Cromp, D., & Taylor, E. F. (2017). Using the Consolidated Framework for Implementation Research (CFIR) to produce actionable findings: A rapid-cycle evaluation approach to improving implementation. *Implementation Science*, *12*, 1–12. https://doi.org/10.1186/s13012-017-0550-7. Medline:28187747

250 Damschroder, L. J., Reardon, C. M., Widerquist, M. A. O., & Lowery, J. (2022). The updated Consolidated Framework for Implementation Research based on user feedback. *Implementation Science: IS*, *17*(1), 75. https://doi.org/10.1186/s13012-022-01245-0. Medline:36309746

251 Knopp, S., Person, B., Ame, S. M., Ali, S. M., Muhsin, J., Juma, S., Khamis, I. S., Rabone, M., Blair, L., Fenwick, A., Mohammed, K. A., & Rollinson, D. (2016). Praziquantel coverage in schools and communities targeted for the elimination of urogenital schistosomiasis in Zanzibar: A cross-sectional

survey. *Parasites & Vectors, 9*(1), 5. https://doi.org/10.1186/s13071-015-1244-0. Medline:26727915

252 Makaula, P., Kayuni, S. A., Mamba, K. C., Bongololo, G., Funsanani, M., Musaya, J., Juziwelo, L. T., & Furu, P. (2022). An assessment of implementation and effectiveness of mass drug administration for prevention and control of schistosomiasis and soil-transmitted helminths in selected southern Malawi districts. *BMC Health Services Research, 22*(1), 517. https://doi.org/10.1186/s12913-022-07925-3. Medline:35439991

253 World Health Organization. (2015). *Mass drug administration to deworm 17 million children underway in Ethiopia*. https://www.afro.who.int/news/mass-drug-administration-deworm-17-million-children-underway-ethiopia

254 Chisha, Y., Zerdo, Z., Asnakew, M., Churko, C., Yihune, M., Teshome, A., Nigussu, N., Seife, F., Getachew, B., & Sileshi, M. (2020). Praziquantel treatment coverage among school age children against schistosomiasis and associated factors in Ethiopia: A cross-sectional survey, 2019. *BMC Infectious Diseases, 20*(1), 872. https://doi.org/10.1186/s12879-020-05519-0. Medline:33225918

255 Federal Ministry of Health of Ethiopia. (2016). *National neglected tropical diseases master plan, 2015/16–2019/20*. World Health Organization Regional Office for Africa. https://www.afro.who.int/publications/second-edition-national-neglected-tropical-diseases-master-plan-ethiopia-2016

256 Hastings, J. (2016). Rumours, riots and the rejection of mass drug administration for the treatment of schistosomiasis in Morogoro, Tanzania. *Journal of Biosocial Science, 48*(S1), S16–S39. https://doi.org/10.1017/S0021932016000018. Medline:27428064

257 Mwandawiro, C. S., Nikolay, B., Kihara, J. H., Ozier, O., Mukoko, D. A., Mwanje, M. T., Hakobyan, A., Pullan, R. L., Brooker, S. J., & Njenga, S. M. (2013). Monitoring and evaluating the impact of national school-based deworming in Kenya: Study design and baseline results. *Parasites & Vectors, 6*(1), 198. https://doi.org/10.1186/1756-3305-6-198. Medline:23829767

258 Kenya Ministry of Health & Kenya Ministry of Education. (2016). *Kenya national school based deworming programme year 4 results (2015–2016)*.. https://files.givewell.org/files/DWDA%202009/DtWI/DtWI_Kenya_National_School_Based_Deworming_Programme_2016.pdf

259 Kenya Ministry of Health & Kenya Ministry of Education. (2017). *Kenya national school-based deworming programme CIFF end-of-project report*. https://files.well.org/files/DWDA%202009/DtWI/Deworm_the_World_Kenya_NSBD_Program_Report_Year_5.pdf

260 Ghana Health Service. (2016). *Master plan for neglected tropical diseases programme, Ghana*. https://espen.afro.who.int/system/files/content/resources/GHANA_NTD_Master_Plan_2016_2020.pdf

261 END NTD in Africa. (2015, February 27). *Train, build trust before treating: Lessons from Ghana's 2014 schistosomiasis MDA*. https://endinafrica.org/news/train-build-trust-before-treating-lessons-from-ghanas-2014-schistosomiasis-mda/

262 Ezezika, O., Daar, A. S., Barber, K., Mabeya, J., Thomas, F., Deadman, J., Wang, D., & Singer, P. A. (2012). Factors influencing agbiotech adoption and development in sub-Saharan Africa. *Nature Biotechnology*, *30*(1), 38–40. https://doi.org/10.1038/nbt.2088. Medline:22231092

263 Karembu, M., Otunge, D., Arujanan, M., Liew, K. C., Choudhary, B., Gaur, K., Choudhary, M. I., Purwantara, B., Panaopio, J., Lapitan, R., Armano, N., Hamid, I. A., Nasiruddin, K., Attahorn, S., Zhang, T., Zhang, H., Navarro, M. J., Tababa, S., & Le, H. (2009). Brief 40 communicating crop biotechnology: stories from stakeholders. *ISAAA*, 197.

264 Karembu, M., Nguthi, F., & Ismail, H. (2009). *Biotech crops in Africa: The final frontier*. ISAAA. https://www.isaaa.org/resources/publications/biotech_crops_in_africa/download/Biotech_Crops_in_Africa-The_Final_Frontier.pdf

265 International Service for the Acquisition of Agri-biotech Applications. (2019). *Global status of commercialized biotech/gm crops in 2019: Biotech crops drive socio economic development and sustainable environment in the new frontier*. https://www.isaaa.org/resources/publications/briefs/55/executivesummary/pdf/B55-ExecSum-English.pdf

266 International Service for the Acquisition of Agri-biotech Applications. (2020). *2020 Accomplishment Report*. https://www.isaaa.org/resources/publications/annualreport/2020/pdf/ISAAA-2020-Accomplishment-Report.pdf

267 International Service for the Acquisition of Agri-biotech Applications. (2017). *Global status of commercialized biotech/gm crops in 2017: Biotech crop adoption surges as economic benefits accumulate in 22 years*. https://www.isaaa.org/resources/publications/briefs/53/download/isaaa-brief-53-2017.pdf

268 International Service for the Acquisition of Agri-biotech Applications. (2016). *Global status of commercialized biotech/GM crops: 2016*. https://www.isaaa.org/resources/publications/briefs/52/executivesummary/pdf/B52-ExecSum-English.pdf

269 Isaac, N. (2020). *Bt cotton in Africa: Role models and lessons learned*. Alliance for Science. https://allianceforscience.cornell.edu/blog/2020/08/bt-cotton-in-africa-role-models-and-lessons-learned/

270 Brookes, G., & Barfoot, P. (2020). GM crops: Global socio-economic and environmental impacts 1996–2018. *GM Crops & Food, 11*(4), 215–241. https://doi.org/10.1080/21645698.2020.1773198

271 Morse, S., Bennett, R., & Ismael, Y. (2005). Bt-cotton boosts the gross margin of small-scale cotton producers in South Africa. *International Journal of Biotechnology, 7*(1–3), 72–83. https://doi.org/10.1504/IJBT.2005.006446

272 Brookes, G., & Barfoot, P. (2008). Global impact of biotech crops: Socio-economic and environmental effects, 1996–2006. *AgBioforum, 11*(1), 21–38.

273 Vitale, J., Glick, H., Greenplate, J., & Traore, O. (2008). The economic impacts of second generation Bt cotton in West Africa: Empirical evidence from Burkina Faso. *International Journal of Biotechnology, 10*(2–3), 167–183. https://doi.org/10.1504/IJBT.2008.018352

274 International Service for the Acquisition of Agri-biotech Applications. (2010). *Global status of commercialized biotech/GM crops: 2010.* https://www.isaaa.org/resources/publications/briefs/42/executivesummary/

275 Juma, C., & Serageldin, I. (2007). *Freedom to innovate: Biotechnology in Africa's development: Report of the High-Level African Panel on Modern Biotechnology.* African Union and New Partnership for Africa's Development. https://www.belfercenter.org/publication/freedom-innovate-biotechnology-africas-development

276 Spielman, D. J., & von Grebmer, K. (2006). Public–Private Partnerships in international agricultural research: An analysis of constraints. *Journal of Technology Transfer, 31*(2), 291–300. https://doi.org/10.1007/s10961-005-6112-1

277 Zheng, J., Roehrich, J. K., & Lewis, M. A. (2008). The dynamics of contractual and relational governance: Evidence from long-term public–private procurement arrangements. *Journal of Purchasing and Supply Management, 14*(1), 43–54. https://doi.org/10.1016/j.pursup.2008.01.004

278 Townsend, S., & Kamau, C. (2020). *Agricultural biotechnology annual.* Foreign Agricultural Service, US Department of Agriculture. https://apps.fas.usda.gov/newgainapi/api/Report/DownloadReportByFileName?fileName=Agricultural%20Biotechnology%20Annual_Nairobi_Kenya_10-20-2020

279 Ezezika, O. (2012). Building effective agbiotech partnerships founded on trust: A summary of the challenges and practices in sub-Saharan Africa. *Agriculture & Food Security, 1*(Suppl. 1), Article S9. https://doi.org/10.1186/2048-7010-1-S1-S9

280 Juma, C. (Ed.). (2012). Fostering innovation through building trust: Lessons from agricultural biotechnology partnerships in Africa. *Agriculture & Food Security, 1*(Suppl. 1). https://agricultureandfoodsecurity.biomedcentral.com/articles/supplements/volume-1-supplement-1

281 Ezezika, O., & Mabeya, J. (2014). Improving communication in agbiotech projects: Moving toward a trust-centered paradigm. *Journal of Applied Communications, 98*(1). https://doi.org/10.4148/1051-0834.1076

282 Ezezika, O., Barber, K., & Daar, A. (2012). The value of trust in biotech crop development: A case study of Bt cotton in Burkina Faso. *Agriculture & Food Security, 1*(Suppl. 1), S2. https://doi.org/10.1186/2048-7010-1-S1-S2

283 Ezezika, O., Lennox, R., & Daar, A. (2012). Strategies for building trust with farmers: The case of Bt maize in South Africa. *Agriculture & Food Security, 1*(1), S3. https://doi.org/10.1186/2048-7010-1-S1-S3

284 Ezezika, O., Deadman, J., Murray, J., Mabeya, J., & Daar, A. (2013). To trust or not to trust: A model for effectively governing public-private partnerships. *AgBioForum, 16*(1), 21–36.

285 Ezezika, O. C., & Oh, J. (2012). What is trust?: Perspectives from farmers and other experts in the field of agriculture in Africa. *Agriculture & Food Security, 1*(1), S1. https://doi.org/10.1186/2048-7010-1-S1-S1

286 Gouse, M., Kristen, J. F., & van Der Walt, W. J. (2008). *Bt cotton and Bt maize: An evaluation of direct and indirect impact on the cotton and maize farming sectors in South Africa*. Department of Agriculture: Directorate BioSafety, Pretoria, South Africa. https://www.gov.uk/research-for-development-outputs/bt-cotton-and-bt-maize-an-evaluation-of-direct-and-indirect-impact-on-the-cotton-and-maize-farming-sectors-in-south-africa

287 Ezezika, O., & Daar, A. (2012). Overcoming barriers to trust in agricultural biotechnology projects: A case study of Bt cowpea in Nigeria. *Agriculture & Food Security, 1*(1), S5. https://doi.org/10.1186/2048-7010-1-S1-S5

288 Ezezika, O., & Daar, A. (2012). Building trust in biotechnology crops in light of the Arab Spring: A case study of Bt maize in Egypt. *Agriculture & Food Security, 1*(1), S4. https://doi.org/10.1186/2048-7010-1-S1-S4

289 Mabeya, J., & Ezezika, O. C. (2012). Unfulfilled farmer expectations: The case of the Insect Resistant Maize for Africa (IRMA) project in Kenya. *Agriculture & Food Security, 1*(1), S6. https://doi.org/10.1186/2048-7010-1-S1-S6

290 Ezezika, O., Mabeya, J., & Daar, A. (2012). Harmonized biosafety regulations are key to trust building in regional agbiotech partnerships: The case of the Bt cotton project in East Africa. *Agriculture & Food Security, 1* (Suppl. 1), S8. https://doi.org/10.1186/2048-7010-1-S1-S8

291 Keetch, D., Ngqaka, A., Akanbi, R., & Mahlanga, P. (2005). Bt maize for small scale farmers: A case study. *African Journal of Food, Agriculture, Nutrition and Development, 4*(13). https://doi.org/10.4314/ajfand.v4i13.71805

292 UNICEF (2016). *Vitamin A supplementation: A statistical snapshot*. https://data.unicef.org/resources/vitamin-supplementation-statistical-snapshot/

293 Aghaji, A. E., Duke, R., & Aghaji, U. C. W. (2019). Inequitable coverage of vitamin A supplementation in Nigeria and implications for childhood blindness. *BMC Public Health, 19*(1), 282. https://doi.org/10.1186/s12889-019-6413-1. Medline:30849959

294 Hasman, A., Imohe, A., Krasevec, J., Moloney, G., & Aguayo, V. M. (2021). COVID-19 caused significant declines in regular vitamin A supplementation for young children in 2020: What is next? *BMJ Global Health, 6*(11), e007507. https://doi.org/10.1136/bmjgh-2021-007507. Medline:34785507

295 Semba, R. D. (2012). On the "discovery" of vitamin A. *Annals of Nutrition & Metabolism, 61*(3), 192–198. https://doi.org/10.1159/000343124. Medline:23798048

296 Soares, M. M., Silva, M. A., Garcia, P. P. C., Silva, da L. S., Costa, da G. D., Araújo, R. M. A., & Cotta, R. M. M. (2019). Effect of vitamin A supplementation: A systematic review. *Ciência & Saúde Coletiva, 24*(3), 827–838. https://doi.org/10.1590/1413-81232018243.07112017. Medline:30892504

297 Underwood, B. A. (1994). Maternal vitamin A status and its importance in infancy and early childhood. *American Journal of Clinical Nutrition, 59*(2), 517S–524S. https://doi.org/10.1093/ajcn/59.2.517S. Medline:8304290

298 World Health Organization. (2009). *Global prevalence of vitamin A deficiency in populations at risk 1995–2005: World Health Organization. global database on vitamin A deficiency*. apps.who.int/iris/bitstream/10665/44110/1/9789241598019_eng.pdf

299 World Health Organization. (1976). *Vitamin A deficiency and xerophthalmia*. https://pdf.usaid.gov/pdf_docs/PNAAD787.pdf

300 Reddy, V. (2002). History of the international vitamin A consultative group 1975–2000. *Journal of Nutrition, 132*(9), 2852S-2856S. https://doi.org/10.1093/jn/132.9.2852S. Medline:12221261

301 Dalmiya, N., & Palmer, A. (2007). *Vitamin A supplementation: A decade of progress*. UNICEF.

302 Ross, D. A. (2002). Recommendations for vitamin A supplementation. *Journal of Nutrition, 132*(9), 2902S–2906S. Medline:12221268

303 Pangaribuan, R., Erhardt, J. G., Scherbaum, V., & Biesalski, H. K. (2003). Vitamin A capsule distribution to control vitamin A deficiency in Indonesia: Effect of supplementation in pre-school children and compliance with the programme. *Public Health Nutrition, 6*(2), 209–216. https://doi.org/10.1079/PHN2002418. Medline:12675964

304 Wirth, J., Petry, N., Tanumihardjo, S., Rogers, L., McLean, E., Greig, A., Garrett, G., Klemm, R., & Rohner, F. (2017). Vitamin A supplementation

programs and country-level evidence of vitamin A deficiency. *Nutrients, 9*(3), 190. https://doi.org/10.3390/nu9030190. Medline:28245571

305 World Health Organization. (2011). *Guideline: Vitamin A supplementation in infants and children 6–59 months of age*. https://iris.who.int/bitstream/handle/10665/44664/9789241501767_eng.pdf

306 Mclaren, D. S. (1964). Xerophthalmia: A neglected problem. *Nutrition Reviews, 22*(10), 289–291. https://doi.org/10.1111/j.1753-4887.1964.tb07483.x. Medline:14221331

307 Sommer, A., Tarwotjo, I., Djunaedi, E., West, K. P., Loeden, A. A., Tilden, R., & Mele, L. (1986). Impact of vitamin A supplementation on childhood mortality. A randomised controlled community trial. *Lancet (London, England), 1*(8491), 1169–1173. https://doi.org/10.1016/s0140-6736(86)91157-8. Medline:2871418

308 Hussey, G. D., & Klein, M. (1990). A randomized, controlled trial of vitamin A in children with severe measles. *New England Journal of Medicine, 323*(3), 160–164. https://doi.org/10.1056/NEJM199007193230304. Medline:2194128

309 Fawzi, W. W., Chalmers, T. C., Herrera, M. G., & Mosteller, F. (1993). Vitamin A supplementation and child mortality: A meta-analysis. *JAMA, 269*(7), 898–903. Medline:8426449

310 Imdad, A., Mayo-Wilson, E., Haykal, M. R., Regan, A., Sidhu, J., Smith, A., & Bhutta, Z. A. (2022). Vitamin A supplementation for preventing morbidity and mortality in children from six months to five years of age. *Cochrane Database of Systematic Reviews*, 3. https://doi.org/10.1002/14651858.CD008524.pub4. Medline:35294044

311 Glasziou, P. P., & Mackerras, D. E. (1993). Vitamin A supplementation in infectious diseases: A meta-analysis. *British Medical Journal, 306*(6874), 366–370. https://doi.org/10.1136/bmj.306.6874.366. Medline:8461682

312 Mayo-Wilson, E., Imdad, A., Herzer, K., Yakoob, M. Y., & Bhutta, Z. A. (2011). Vitamin A supplements for preventing mortality, illness, and blindness in children aged under 5: Systematic review and meta-analysis. *BMJ, 343*, d5094. https://doi.org/10.1136/bmj.d5094. Medline:21868478

313 World Bank. (2020). *Mortality rate, under-5 (per 1,000 live births) – Sub-Saharan Africa*. https://data.worldbank.org/indicator/SH.DYN.MORT?locations=ZG

314 Klemm, R. D. W., Palmer, A. C., Greig, A., Engle-Stone, R., & Dalmiya, N. (2016). A changing landscape for vitamin A programs: Implications for optimal intervention packages, program monitoring, and safety. *Food and Nutrition Bulletin, 37*(2 Suppl.), S75–S86. https://doi.org/10.1177/0379572116630481. Medline:27004480

315 Ahmed, F. (1999). Vitamin A deficiency in Bangladesh: A review and recommendations for improvement. *Public Health Nutrition*, *2*(1), 1–14. https://doi.org/10.1017/S1368980099000014. Medline:10452726

316 McLean, E., Klemm, R., Subramaniam, H., & Greig, A. (2020). Refocusing vitamin A supplementation programmes to reach the most vulnerable. *BMJ Global Health*, *5*(7), e001997. https://doi.org/10.1136/bmjgh-2019-001997. Medline:32718947

317 McLean, E., White, J., Krasevec, J., Kupka, R., & UNICEF. (2018). *Coverage at a crossroads: New directions for vitamin A supplementation programmes.* UNICEF. https://www.unicef.org/media/48031/file/vitamin-a-report-eng.pdf

318 UNICEF. (2019). *Monitoring the situation of children and women – vitamin A supplementation interactive dashboard.*

319 Nutrition International. (2021, June 1). *Nutrition International to lead vitamin A supplementation catch-up efforts for children in Africa as part of Canada's response to COVID-19.* [Press release]. https://reliefweb.int/report/world/nutrition-international-lead-vitamin-supplementation-catch-efforts-children-africa-part

320 Thorne-Lyman, A. L., Parajuli, K., Paudyal, N., Chitekwe, S., Shrestha, R., Manandhar, D. L., & West Jr, K. P. (2022). To see, hear, and live: 25 years of the vitamin A programme in Nepal. *Maternal & Child Nutrition*, *18*(S1), e12954. https://doi.org/10.1111/mcn.12954. Medline:32108438

321 Coutsoudis, A., Broughton, M., & Coovadia, H. M. (1991). Vitamin A supplementation reduces measles morbidity in young African children: A randomized, placebo-controlled, double-blind trial. *American Journal of Clinical Nutrition*, *54*(5), 890–895. https://doi.org/10.1093/ajcn/54.5.890. Medline:1951162

322 SanJoaquin, M. A., & Molyneux, M. E. (2009). Malaria and vitamin A deficiency in African children: A vicious circle? *Malaria Journal*, *8*, 134. https://doi.org/10.1186/1475-2875-8-134. Medline:19534807

323 Roser, M., & Ritchie, H. (2019). *Malaria*. Our World in Data. https://ourworldindata.org/malaria

324 Baye, K., Laillou, A., Seyoum, Y., Zvandaziva, C., Chimanya, K., & Nyawo, M. (2022). Estimates of child mortality reductions attributed to vitamin A supplementation in sub-Saharan Africa: Scale up, scale back, or refocus? *American Journal of Clinical Nutrition*, *116*(2), 426–434. https://doi.org/10.1093/ajcn/nqac082. Medline:35380631

325 UNICEF. (n.d.). *Vitamin A supplementation coverage rate (% of children ages 6–59 months)—Sub-Saharan Africa.* Retrieved October 9, 2022, from https://data.worldbank.org/indicator/SN.ITK.VITA.ZS?locations=ZG&most_recent_value_desc=false

326 Kannan, A., Tsoi, D., Xie, Y., Horst, C., Collins, J., & Flaxman, A. (2022). Cost-effectiveness of vitamin A supplementation among children in three sub-Saharan African countries: An individual-based simulation model using estimates from Global Burden of Disease 2019. *PLOS ONE*, *17*(4), e0266495. https://doi.org/10.1371/journal.pone.0266495. Medline:35390077

327 Abessolo, F. O., Kuissi, E., Nguele, J. C., Lémamy, G. J., Ndong, Z., & Ngou-Milama, E. (2009). Vitamin A in Gabonese children not receiving supplements: Relation to ocular and nutritional diseases. *Sante (Montrouge, France)*, *19*(1), 29–33. https://doi.org/10.1684/san.2009.0142. Medline:19801349

328 Nutrition International. (2021, August 30). *Insight from the frontlines: why is a vitamin A catch-up initiative needed now?* https://www.nutritionintl.org/news/all-field-stories/why-is-a-vitamin-a-catch-up-initiative-needed-covid-19/

329 Oyunga, M., Okeyo, D., & Grant, F. (2016). Awareness in the context of prevalence of vitamin A deficiency among households in Western Kenya using a cross-sectional study. *Food and Nutrition Sciences*, *4*(3), 55–64. https://doi.org/10.11648/j.jfns.20160403.13

330 Berde, A. S., Bester, P., & Kruger, I. M. (2019). Coverage and factors associated with vitamin A supplementation among children aged 6–59 months in twenty-three sub-Saharan African countries. *Public Health Nutrition*, *22*(10), 1770–1776. https://doi.org/10.1017/S1368980018004056. Medline:30755287

331 Dube, W. G., Makoni, T., Nyadzayo, T. K., & Covic, N. M. (2014). A strategy for scaling up vitamin A supplementation for young children in a remote rural setting in Zimbabwe. *South African Journal of Child Health*, *8*(2), 64–67. https://doi.org/10.7196/SAJCH.618

332 Bruins, M., & Kraemer, K. (2013). Public health programmes for vitamin A deficiency control. *Community Eye Health*, *26*(84), 69–70. Medline:24782583

333 Ayoya, M. A., Bendech, M. A., Baker, S. K., Ouattara, F., Diané, K. A., Mahy, L., Nichols, L., Touré, A., & Franco, C. (2007). Determinants of high vitamin A supplementation coverage among pre-school children in Mali: The National Nutrition Weeks experience. *Public Health Nutrition*, *10*(11), 1241–1246. https://doi.org/10.1017/S1368980007687138. Medline:17381941

334 Demissie, T., Haider, J., & Tibeb, H. N. (2003). Process evaluation of an EPI-integrated vitamin A capsule delivery programme in KAT zone, southern Ethiopia. *South African Journal of Clinical Nutrition*, *16*(1), 5.

335 du Plessis, L. M., Najaar, B., Koornhof, H. E., Labaarios, D., Petersen, L., Hendricks, M. A., & Kidd, M. (2007). Evaluation of the implementation

of the vitamin A supplementation programme in the Boland/Overberg region of the Western Cape Province. *South African Journal of Clinical Nutrition, 20*, 126–132. https://doi.org/10.1080/16070658.2007.11734139

336 Luthringer, C. L., Rowe, L. A., Vossenaar, M., & Garrett, G. S. (2015). Regulatory monitoring of fortified foods: Identifying barriers and good practices. *Global Health: Science and Practice, 3*(3), 446–461. https://doi.org/10.9745/GHSP-D-15-00171. Medline:26374804

337 Neidecker-Gonzales, O., Nestel, P., & Bouis, H. (2007). Estimating the global costs of vitamin A capsule supplementation: A review of the literature. *Food and Nutrition Bulletin, 28*(3), 307–316. https://doi.org/10.1177/156482650702800307. Medline:17974364

338 Lyatuu, M. B., Mkumbwa, T., Stevenson, R., Isidro, M., Modaha, F., Katcher, H., & Dhillon, C. N. (2016). Planning and budgeting for nutrition programs in Tanzania: Lessons learned from the national vitamin A supplementation program. *International Journal of Health Policy and Management, 5*(10), 583–588. https://doi.org/10.15171/ijhpm.2016.46. Medline:27694649

339 Oiye, S., Safari, N., Anyango, J., Arimi, C., Nyawa, B., Kimeu, M., Odinde, J., Kambona, O., Kahindi, R., & Mutisya, R. (2019). Programmatic implications of some vitamin A supplementation and deworming determinants among children aged 6–59 months in resource-poor rural Kenya. *Pan African Medical Journal, 32*, 96. https://doi.org/10.11604/pamj.2019.32.96.17221. Medline:31231453

340 Fiedler, J. L., & Lividini, K. (2014). Managing the vitamin A program portfolio: A case study of Zambia, 2013–2042. *Food and Nutrition Bulletin, 35*(1), 105–125. https://doi.org/10.1177/156482651403500112. Medline:24791584

341 Fiedler, J. L. (2000). The Nepal National Vitamin A Program: Prototype to emulate or donor enclave? *Health Policy and Planning, 15*(2), 145–156. https://doi.org/10.1093/heapol/15.2.145

342 de Wagt, A. (2001). Vitamin A deficiency control programs in Eastern and Southern Africa: A Unicef perspective. *Food and Nutrition Bulletin, 22*(4), 352–356. https://doi.org/10.1177/156482650102200402

343 Hill, Z., Kirkwood, B., Kendall, C., Adjei, E., Arthur, P., & Agyemang, C. T. (2007). Factors that affect the adoption and maintenance of weekly vitamin A supplementation among women in Ghana. *Public Health Nutrition, 10*(8), 827–833. https://doi.org/10.1017/S1368980007382554. Medline:17381927

344 Hendricks, M., Beardsley, J., Bourne, L., Mzamo, B., & Golden, B. (2007). Are opportunities for vitamin A supplementation being utilised at primary healthcare clinics in the Western Cape Province of South Africa? *Public Health Nutrition, 10*(10), 1082–1088. https://doi.org/10.1017/S1368980007699522. Medline:17381904

345 Nyhus Dhillon, C., Subramaniam, H., Mulokozi, G., Rambeloson, Z., & Klemm, R. (2013). Overestimation of vitamin A supplementation coverage from district Tally Sheets demonstrates the importance of population-based surveys for program improvement: Lessons from Tanzania. *PLoS ONE, 8*(3), e58629. https://doi.org/10.1371/journal.pone.0058629. Medline:23536804

346 Mahajan, H., Srivastav, S., & Mukherjee, S. (2016). Coverage of vitamin A supplementation among under-five children in an urban resettlement colony of district Gautam-Budh Nagar, Uttar Pradesh. *International Journal of Medical Science and Public Health, 5*(7), 1328. https://doi.org/10.5455/ijmsph.2016.11092015191

347 Popa, A. D., Niță, O., Graur, L. I., Popescu, R. M., Botnariu, G. E., Mihalache, L., & Graur, M. (2013). Nutritional knowledge as a determinant of vitamin and mineral supplementation during pregnancy. *BMC Public Health, 13*(1), 1105. https://doi.org/10.1186/1471-2458-13-1105. Medline:24289203

348 Kamau, M., Mirie, W., Kimani, S., & Mugoya, I. (2019). Effect of community-based health education on knowledge and attitude towards iron and folic acid supplementation among pregnant women in Kiambu County, Kenya: A quasi-experimental study. *PLOS ONE, 14*(11), e0224361. https://doi.org/10.1371/journal.pone.0224361. Medline:31765422

349 Vonasek, B. J., Bajunirwe, F., Jacobson, L. E., Twesigye, L., Dahm, J., Grant, M. J., Sethi, A. K., & Conway, J. H. (2016). Do maternal knowledge and attitudes towards childhood immunizations in rural Uganda correlate with complete childhood vaccination? *PloS One, 11*(2), e0150131. https://doi.org/10.1371/journal.pone.0150131. Medline:26918890

350 Semba, R. D., de Pee, S., Sun, K., Bloem, M. W., & Raju, V. K. (2008). Coverage of the national vitamin A supplementation program in Ethiopia. *Journal of Tropical Pediatrics, 54*(2), 141–144. https://doi.org/10.1093/tropej/fmm095. Medline:18304953

351 Adamu, M., & Muhammad, N. (2016). Assessment of vitamin A supplementation coverage and associated barriers in Sokoto State, Nigeria. *Annals of Nigerian Medicine, 10*(1), 16. https://doi.org/10.4103/0331-3131.189803

352 Agrawal, S., & Agrawal, P. (2013). Vitamin A supplementation among children in India: Does their socioeconomic status and the economic and social development status of their state of residence make a difference? *International Journal of Medicine and Public Health, 3*(1), 48. https://doi.org/10.4103/2230-8598.109322. Medline:25729705

353 Nguyen, A. M., Grover, D. S., Sun, K., Raju, V. K., Semba, R. D., & Schaumerg, D. A. (2012). Coverage of the vitamin A supplementation programme for child survival in Nepal: Success and challenges.

Paediatrics and International Child Health, 32(4), 233–238. https://doi.org/10.1179/2046905512Y.0000000037. Medline:23164298

354 Haile, D., Biadgilign, S., & Azage, M. (2015). Differentials in vitamin A supplementation among preschool-aged children in Ethiopia: Evidence from the 2011 Ethiopian demographic and health Survey. *Public Health, 129*(6), 748–754. https://doi.org/10.1016/j.puhe.2015.03.001. Medline:25982948

355 Tandon, B. N. (1981). A coordinated approach to children's health in India. *Lancet (London, England), 1*(8221), 650–653. Medline:6110873

356 Thapa, S., Choe, M. K., & Retherford, R. D. (2005). Effects of vitamin A supplementation on child mortality: Evidence from Nepal's 2001 Demographic and Health Survey. *Tropical Medicine and International Health, 10*(8), 782–789. https://doi.org/10.1111/j.1365-3156.2005.01448.x. Medline:16045465

357 Rah, J. H., Houston, R., Mohapatra, B. D., Kumar, S. S., Saiyed, F., Bhattacharjee, S., & Aguayo, V. M. (2014). A review of the vitamin A supplementation program in India: Reasons for success in the states of Bihar and Odisha. *Food and Nutrition Bulletin, 35*(2), 203–210. https://doi.org/10.1177/156482651403500207. Medline:25076768

358 Gorstein, J., Bhaskaram, P., Khanum, S., Hossaini, R., Balakrishna, N., Goodman, T. S., deBenoist, B., & Krishnaswamy, K. (2003). Safety and impact of vitamin A supplementation delivered with oral polio vaccine as part of the immunization campaign in Orissa, India. *Food and Nutrition Bulletin, 24*(4), 319–331. https://doi.org/10.1177/156482650302400402. Medline:14870619

359 Pedro, M. R. A., Madriaga, J. R., Barba, C. V. C., Habito, R. C. F., Gana, A. E., Deitchler, M., & Mason, J. B. (2004). The National Vitamin A Supplementation Program and subclinical vitamin A deficiency among preschool children in the Philippines. *Food and Nutrition Bulletin, 25*(4), 319–329. https://doi.org/10.1177/156482650402500401. Medline:15646309

360 Aguayo, V. M., Baker, S. K., Crespin, X., Hamani, H., & MamadoulTaïbou, A. (2005). Maintaining high vitamin A supplementation coverage in children: Lessons from Niger. *Food and Nutrition Bulletin, 26*(1), 26–31. https://doi.org/10.1177/156482650502600103. Medline:15810796

361 Ching, P., Birmingham, M., Goodman, T. S., Sutter, R., & Loevinsohn, B. (2000). Childhood mortality impact and costs of integrating vitamin A supplementation into immunization campaigns. *American Journal of Public Health, 90*(10), 1526–1529. https://doi.org/10.2105/AJPH.90.10.1526. Medline:11029982

362 Benn, C. S., Rodrigues, A., Yazdanbakhsh, M., Fisker, A. B., Ravn, H., Whittle, H., & Aaby, P. (2009). The effect of high-dose vitamin A supplementation administered with BCG vaccine at birth may be

modified by subsequent DTP vaccination. *Vaccine, 27*(21), 2891–2898. https://doi.org/10.1016/j.vaccine.2009.02.080. Medline:19428899

363 Masanja, H., Schellenberg, J. A., Mshinda, H. M., Shekar, M., Mugyabuso, J. K., Ndossi, G. D., & de Savigny, D. (2006). Vitamin A supplementation in Tanzania: The impact of a change in programmatic delivery strategy on coverage. *BMC Health Services Research, 6*(1), 142. https://doi.org/10.1186/1472-6963-6-142. Medline:17078872

364 Deitchler, M., Mathys, E., Mason, J., Winichagoon, P., & Tuazon, M. A. (2004). Lessons from successful micronutrient programs part II: Program implementation. *Food and Nutrition Bulletin, 25*(1), 30–52. https://doi.org/10.1177/156482650402500103. Medline:18018367

365 Grover, D. S., De Pee, S., Sun, K., Raju, V. K., Bloem, M. W., & Semba, R. D. (2008). Vitamin A supplementation in Cambodia: Program coverage and association with greater maternal formal education. *Pacific Journal of Clinical Nutrition, 17*(3), 446–450. Medline:18818165

366 Khan, N. C., Khoi, H. H., Giay, T., Nhan, N. T., Nhan, N. T., Dung, N. C., Thang, H. V., Dien, D. N., & Luy, H. T. (2002). Control of vitamin A deficiency in Vietnam: Achievements and future orientation. *Food and Nutrition Bulletin, 23*(2), 133–142. https://doi.org/10.1177/156482650202300202. Medline:12094663

367 Pangaribuan, R. (2004). Socioeconomic and familial characteristics influence caretakers' adherence to the periodic vitamin A capsule supplementation program in Central Java, Indonesia. *Journal of Tropical Pediatrics, 50*(3), 143–148. https://doi.org/10.1093/tropej/50.3.143. Medline:15233189

368 Istepanian, R., Laxminarayan, S., & Pattichis, C. (2006). Ubiquitous m-health systems and the convergence towards 4G mobile technologies. In *M-health: Emerging mobile health systems* (p. 3). Springer.

369 Wachter, R. (2015). *The digital doctor: Hope, hype, and harm at the dawn of medicine's computer age*. McGraw-Hill.

370 Liu, P., Astudillo, K., Velez, D., Kelley, L., Cobbs-Lomax, D., & Spatz, E. S. (2020). Use of mobile health applications in low-income populations: A prospective study of facilitators and barriers. *Circulation: Cardiovascular Quality and Outcomes, 13*(9), e007031. https://doi.org/10.1161/CIRCOUTCOMES.120.007031. Medline:32885681

371 World Health Organization. (2018). *mHealth: Use of appropriate digital technologies for public health. Seventy-First World Health Assembly, A71/20*. https://apps.who.int/gb/ebwha/pdf_files/WHA71/A71_20-en.pdf

372 Fiordelli, M., Diviani, N., & Schulz, P. J. (2013). Mapping mhealth research: A decade of evolution. *Journal of Medical Internet Research, 15*(5). https://doi.org/10.2196/jmir.2430. Medline:23697600

373 Boogerd, E. A., Arts, T., Engelen, L. J., & van De Belt, T. H. (2015). "What is eHealth": Time for an update? *JMIR Research Protocols, 4*(1), Article e4065. https://doi.org/10.2196/resprot.4065. Medline:25768939

374 World Bank. (2012). *2012 Information and communications for development: Maximizing mobile.* https://hdl.handle.net/10986/11958

375 Allen, L. N., & Christie, G. P. (2016). The emergence of personalized health technology. *Journal of Medical Internet Research, 18*(5), e99. https://doi.org/10.2196/jmir.5357. Medline:27165944

376 Lee, S., Cho, Y., & Kim, S.-Y. (2017). Mapping mHealth (mobile health) and mobile penetrations in sub-Saharan Africa for strategic regional collaboration in mHealth scale-up: An application of exploratory spatial data analysis. *Globalization and Health, 13*(1), 63. https://doi.org/10.1186/s12992-017-0286-9. Medline:28830540

377 Oh, H., Rizo, C., Enkin, M., & Jadad, A. (2005). What is eHealth (3): A systematic review of published definitions. *Journal of Medical Internet Research, 7*(1), e1. https://doi.org/10.2196/jmir.7.1.e1. Medline:15829471

378 Della Mea, V. (2001). What is e-Health (2): The death of telemedicine? *Journal of Medical Internet Research, 3*(2), e22. https://doi.org/10.2196/jmir.3.2.e22. Medline:11720964

379 Ginsberg, J., Mohebbi, M. H., Patel, R. S., Brammer, L., Smolinski, M. S., & Brilliant, L. (2009). Detecting influenza epidemics using search engine query data. *Nature, 457*(7232), 1012–1014. https://doi.org/10.1038/nature07634. Medline:19020500

380 Yoneki, E. (2011). *FluPhone study: Virtual disease spread using haggle.* Proceedings of the Annual International Conference on Mobile Computing and Networking, MOBICOM, 65–66. https://doi.org/10.1145/2030652.2030672

381 Innovation Eye (2020). *Global mHealth industry landscape overview 2020.* https://analytics.dkv.global/global-mhealth-industry-2020/report.pdf

382 FrontlineSMS. (2012). *Mobile and development intelligence.* https://www.gsma.com/solutions-and-impact/connectivity-for-good/mobile-for-development/wp-content/uploads/2016/02/Case_Study_-FrontlineSMS_.pdf

383 Mwendwa, P. (2016). Assessing the fit of RapidSMS for maternal and newborn health: Perspectives of community health workers in rural Rwanda. *Development in Practice, 26*(1), 38–51. https://doi.org/10.1080/09614524.2016.1112769

384 RapidSMS. (2016). *Tracking the first 1000 days of life, preventing unnecessary mother and newborn deaths.* https://lib.digitalsquare.io/server/api/core/bitstreams/c7ccda66-470d-4208-88ac-9a4592df1151/content

385 Datadyne. (n.d.). *EpiSurveyor brief.* http://www.africanstrategies4health.org/uploads/1/3/5/3/13538666/episurveyormagpi.pdf

386 Seebregts, C., Barron, P., Tanna, G., Benjamin, P., & Fogwill, T. (2016). MomConnect: An exemplar implementation of the Health Normative Standards Framework in South Africa. *South African Health Review*, 2016(1), 125–135.

387 United Nations Development Programme. (2021). *Vula Mobile. SDG Finance Geneva Summit*. https://s3.amazonaws.com/bizzabo.users.files/131692/222993/5669651/Health_Vula_April12.pdf

388 GiftedMom. (n.d.). *Using mobile channels to democratise and reinvent access to maternal healthcare in Francophone Africa*. https://www.gsma.com/solutions-and-impact/connectivity-for-good/mobile-for-development/wp-content/uploads/2019/08/GiftedMom-Using-mobile-channels-to-democratise-and-reinvent-access-to-maternal-healthcare-in-Francophone-Africa_SINGLE.pdf

389 World Health Organization. (2016). *Global diffusion of eHealth: Making universal health coverage achievable: Report of the third global survey on eHealth*. https://www.who.int/publications/i/item/9789241511780

390 Noriega, S., & Eveslage, B. (2022). *Digital health landscape report: Promise 2021 digital health landscape report for introduction of new HIV prevention products in Africa*. from: https://www.fhi360.org/wp-content/uploads/drupal/documents/resource-going-online-digital-health-landscaping-report.pdf

391 Ezezika, O., Varatharajan, C., Racine, S., & Ameyaw, E. (2021). The implementation of a maternal mHealth project in South Africa: Lessons for taking mHealth innovations to scale. *African Journal of Science, Technology, Innovation and Development*. https://doi.org/10.1080/20421338.2021.1985946

392 Ruton, H., Musabyimana, A., Grépin, K., Ngenzi, J., Nzabonimana, E., & Law, M. R. (2016). *Evaluating the impact of RapidSMS: Final report*. International Household Survey Network. https://catalog.ihsn.org/citations/80749

393 Cable.co.uk. (2022). *Worldwide mobile data pricing 2022*. https://www.cable.co.uk/mobiles/worldwide-data-pricing/2022/press_release_global_mobile_data_pricing_study_2022.pdf

394 UNICEF. (2015). *Nutritional surveillance in Malawi*. https://www.unicef.org/innovation/stories/nutritional-surveillance-malawi

395 Northrop, W. (2016, August 13). Cameroonian creates life-saving app "Gifted Mom." *BORGEN*. https://www.borgenmagazine.com/cameroonian-entrepreneur-app-gifted-mom/

396 Siering, H. (n.d.). *GiftedMom: How a simple SMS could save your life in Cameroon*. Reset. https://en.reset.org/giftedmom-sms-service-fuer-schwangere-und-muetter-12282016/

397 Parfitt, B. (2011). *Using SMS to help people with HIV in rural Kenya*. FrontlineSMS. https://www.frontlinesms.com/blog/2011/11/15/using-sms-to-help-people-with-hiv-in-rural-kenya

398 Merwe, E. van der, & Grobbelaar, S. (2018). Systemic policy instruments for inclusive innovation systems: Case study of a maternal mHealth project in South Africa. *African Journal of Science, Technology, Innovation and Development, 10*(6), 665–682. https://doi.org/10.1080/20421338.2018.1491678

399 Seebregts, C., Dane, P., Parsons, A. N., Fogwill, T., Rogers, D., Bekker, M., Shaw, V., & Barron, P. (2018). Designing for scale: Optimising the health information system architecture for mobile maternal health messaging in South Africa (MomConnect). *BMJ Global Health, 3*(Suppl. 2), e000563. https://doi.org/10.1136/bmjgh-2017-000563. Medline:29713506

400 van Dyk, L. (2014). A review of telehealth service implementation frameworks. *International Journal of Environmental Research and Public Health, 11*(2), 1279–1298. https://doi.org/10.3390/ijerph110201279. Medline:24464237

401 Holly, L., Smith, R. D., Ndili, N., Franz, C., & Stevens, E. A. G. (2022). A review of digital health strategies in 10 countries with young populations: Do they serve the health and wellbeing of children and youth in a digital age? *Frontiers in Digital Health, 4*, 817810. https://doi.org/10.3389/fdgth.2022.817810. Medline:35373182

402 Vula Mobile. (n.d.).*Legal & compliance*. https://www.vulamobile.com/legal-and-compliance

403 *Ethical rules of conduct for practitioners registered under the health professions Act 1974*. (1974). BN 26, G. 36183 (c.i.o 1 March 2013). http://www.saflii.org/za/legis/consol_reg/erocfpruthpa1974803/

404 Kubheka, B. (2017). Ethical and legal perspectives on the medical practitioners' use of social media. *South African Medical Journal, 107*(5), Article 5. https://doi.org/10.7196/SAMJ.2017.v107i5.12047. Medline:28492116

405 Steyn, L., Mash, R. J., & Hendricks, G. (2022). Use of the Vula App to refer patients in the West Coast District: A descriptive exploratory qualitative study. *South African Family Practice, 64*(1), 5491. https://doi.org/10.4102/safp.v64i1.5491. Medline:35532127

406 World Health Organization. (2023, December 4). *Malaria*. https://www.who.int/news-room/fact-sheets/detail/malaria

407 Sinka, M. E. (2013, July 24). *Global distribution of the dominant vector species of malaria*. IntechOpen. https://www.intechopen.com/chapters/43624

408 Fauci, A. S. (n.d.). *Commentary: Yes, we can eradicate malaria*. CNN. Retrieved 25 March 2024, from https://www.cnn.com/2009/HEALTH/conditions/04/25/fauci.malaria/

409 Pryce, J., Richardson, M., & Lengeler, C. (2018). Insecticide-treated nets for preventing malaria. *Cochrane Database of Systematic Reviews, 2018*(11), CD000363. https://doi.org/10.1002/14651858.CD000363.pub3. Medline:30398672

410 Wetzler, E. A., Park, C., Arroz, J. A. H., Chande, M., Mussambala, F., & Candrinho, B. (2022). Impact of mass distribution of insecticide-treated nets in Mozambique, 2012 to 2025: Estimates of child lives saved using the Lives Saved Tool. *PLOS Global Public Health*, 2(4), e0000248. https://doi.org/10.1371/journal.pgph.0000248. Medline:36962318

411 Abdulla, S., Schellenberg, J. A., Nathan, R., Mukasa, O., Marchant, T., Smith, T., Tanner, M., & Lengeler, C. (2001). Impact on malaria morbidity of a programme supplying insecticide treated nets in children aged under 2 years in Tanzania: Community cross sectional study. *BMJ : British Medical Journal*, *322*(7281), 270–273. https://doi.org/10.1136/bmj.322.7281.270. Medline:11157527

412 Lindsay, S. W., & Gibson, M. E. (1988). Bednets revisited – Old idea, new angle. *Parasitology Today (Personal Ed.)*, *4*(10), 270–272. https://doi.org/10.1016/0169-4758(88)90017-8. Medline:15462999

413 Russell, P. F. (1955). *Man's mastery of malaria*. Internet Archive. http://archive.org/details/in.ernet.dli.2015.549635

414 MacCormack, C. P. (1984). Human ecology and behaviour in malaria control in tropical Africa. *Bulletin of the World Health Organization*, *62*(Suppl.), 81–87. Medline:6335685

415 Nájera, J. A., González-Silva, M., & Alonso, P. L. (2011). Some lessons for the future from the global malaria eradication programme (1955–1969). *PLoS Medicine*, *8*(1), e1000412. https://doi.org/10.1371/journal.pmed.1000412. Medline:21311585

416 Sadasivaiah, S., Tozan, Y., & Breman, J. G. (2007). Dichlorodiphenyltrichloroethane (DDT) for indoor residual spraying in Africa: How can it be used for malaria control? In J. G. Breman, M. S. Alilio, & N. J. White (Eds.), *Defining and Defeating the Intolerable Burden of Malaria III: Progress and Perspectives: Supplement to Volume 77(6) of American Journal of Tropical Medicine and Hygiene*. American Society of Tropical Medicine and Hygiene. https://www.ncbi.nlm.nih.gov/books/NBK1724/

417 Harper, P. A., Lisansky, E. T., & Sasse, B. E. (1947). *Malaria and other insect-borne diseases in the South Pacific campaign, 1942–1945*. National Library of Medicine. https://collections.nlm.nih.gov/catalog/nlm:nlmuid-101583859-bk

418 Darriet, F., Robert, V., Vien, N. T., Carnevale, P., & Organization, W. H. (1984). *Evaluation of the efficacy of Permethrin impregnated intact and perforated mosquito nets against vectors of malaria (WHO/MAL/84.1008)*. Article WHO/MAL/84.1008. World Health Organization. https://iris.who.int/handle/10665/65908

419 World Health Organization. (1993). *A global strategy for malaria control*. https://iris.who.int/handle/10665/41785

420 Malaria Consortium. (n.d.). *Malaria prevention*. https://www.malariaconsortium.org/pages/malaria_control.htm

421 VanNoy, B. N. (n.d.). *Climate change impacts on malaria transmission in West African countries*. PressBooks. https://ohiostate.pressbooks.pub/sciencebitesvolume2/chapter/4-3-climate-change-impacts-on-malaria-transmission-in-west-african-countries/

422 Miller, J. M., Korenromp, E. L., Nahlen, B. L., & W Steketee, R. (2007). Estimating the number of insecticide-treated nets required by African households to reach continent-wide malaria coverage targets. *JAMA, 297*(20), 2241–2250. https://doi.org/10.1001/jama.297.20.2241. Medline:17519414

423 Roll Back Malaria, World Health Organization, & UNICEF. (2005, November 18). *World malaria report 2005*. https://www.who.int/publications-detail-redirect/9241593199

424 Thwing, J., Hochberg, N., Vanden Eng, J., Issifi, S., Eliades, M. J., Minkoulou, E., Wolkon, A., Gado, H., Ibrahim, O., Newman, R. D., & Lama, M. (2008). Insecticide-treated net ownership and usage in Niger after a nationwide integrated campaign. *Tropical Medicine & International Health: TM & IH, 13*(6), 827–834. https://doi.org/10.1111/j.1365-3156.2008.02070.x. Medline:18384476

425 Centers for Disease Control and Prevention. (2005, October 7). *Distribution of insecticide-treated bednets during an integrated nationwide immunization campaign – Togo, West Africa, December 2004*. https://www.cdc.gov/mmwr/preview/mmwrhtml/mm5439a6.htm

426 World Health Organization. (2018). *World malaria report 2018*. https://www.who.int/publications-detail-redirect/9789241565653

427 World Health Organization. (n.d.). *Malaria*. Regional Office for Africa. https://www.afro.who.int/health-topics/malaria

428 Atta, H., & Zamani, G. (2008). *The progress of Roll Back Malaria in the Eastern Mediterranean Region over the past decade*. World Health Organization Regional Office for the Eastern Mediterranean. http://www.emro.who.int/emhj-volume-14-2008/volume-14-supplement/the-progress-of-roll-back-malaria-in-the-eastern-mediterranean-region-over-the-past-decade.html

429 Yamey, G. (2000). African heads of state promise action against malaria. *BMJ (Clinical Research Ed.), 320*(7244), 1228. https://doi.org/10.1136/bmj.320.7244.1228. Medline:10797028

430 World Health Organization & UNICEF. (2003). *The Africa malaria report 2003*. https://iris.who.int/handle/10665/67869

431 Hanson, K., Marchant, T., Nathan, R., Mponda, H., Jones, C., Bruce, J., Mshinda, H., & Schellenberg, J. A. (2009). Household ownership and use of insecticide treated nets among target groups after implementation

of a national voucher programme in the United Republic of Tanzania: Plausibility study using three annual cross sectional household surveys. *BMJ*, *339*, b2434. https://doi.org/10.1136/bmj.b2434. Medline:19574316

432 Bonner, K., Mwita, A., McElroy, P. D., Omari, S., Mzava, A., Lengeler, C., Kaspar, N., Nathan, R., Ngegba, J., Mtung'e, R., & Brown, N. (2011). Design, implementation and evaluation of a national campaign to distribute nine million free LLINs to children under five years of age in Tanzania. *Malaria Journal*, *10*, 73. https://doi.org/10.1186/1475-2875-10-73. Medline:21453519

433 Abdulahi, A. A., Van Zyl-Schalekamp, C., Senaka, A., Abdullahi, A. A., & Seneka, A. (2013). Perceived threat of malaria and the use of insecticide treated bed nets in Nigeria. *African Sociological Review/Revue Africaine de Sociologie*, *17*(1), 25–44.

434 Baume, C. A., & Marin, M. C. (2008). Gains in awareness, ownership and use of insecticide-treated nets in Nigeria, Senegal, Uganda and Zambia. *Malaria Journal*, *7*, 153. https://doi.org/10.1186/1475-2875-7-153. Medline:18687145

435 Federal Republic of Nigeria. (2014). *National malaria strategic plan 2014–2020*.

436 Onyeneho, N. G. (2013). Sleeping under insecticide-treated nets to prevent malaria in Nigeria: What do we know? *Journal of Health, Population, and Nutrition*, *31*(2), 243–251. https://doi.org/10.3329/jhpn.v31i2.16389. Medline:23930343

437 Roll Back Malaria Partnership. (2012). *Focus on Nigeria: Progress & impact series*. chrome-extension://efaidnbmnnnibpcajpcglclefindmkaj/https://www.mmv.org/sites/default/files/uploads/docs/publications/RBM_Nigeria_3.pdf

438 Attah, S. (2022, February 15). *Nasarawa commences distribution of over 2m treated mosquito nets*. Businessday NG. https://businessday.ng/news/article/nasarawa-commences-distribution-of-over-2m-treated-mosquito-nets/

439 Ahorlu, C. S., Adongo, P., Koenker, H., Zigirumugabe, S., Sika-Bright, S., Koka, E., Tabong, P. T.-N., Piccinini, D., Segbaya, S., Olapeju, B., & Monroe, A. (2019). Understanding the gap between access and use: A qualitative study on barriers and facilitators to insecticide-treated net use in Ghana. *Malaria Journal*, *18*(1), 417. https://doi.org/10.1186/s12936-019-3051-0. Medline:31831004

440 Kim, S., Piccinini, D., Mensah, E., & Lynch, M. (2019). Using a human-centered design approach to determine consumer preferences for long-lasting insecticidal nets in Ghana. *Global Health: Science and Practice*, *7*(2), 160–170. https://doi.org/10.9745/GHSP-D-18-00284. Medline:31249018

441 Pulford, J., Hetzel, M. W., Bryant, M., Siba, P. M., & Mueller, I. (2011). Reported reasons for not using a mosquito net when one is available: A

review of the published literature. *Malaria Journal, 10*, 83. https://doi.org/10.1186/1475-2875-10-83. Medline:21477376

442 Desmon, S. (2019, June 27). *"Why don't we ask people what they want?:" Bed net use in Ghana*. Johns Hopkins Center for Communication Programs. https://ccp.jhu.edu/2019/06/27/human-centered-design-bed-mosquito-net/

443 Alfonso, Y. N., Lynch, M., Mensah, E., Piccinini, D., & Bishai, D. (2020). Willingness-to-pay for long-lasting insecticide-treated bed nets: A discrete choice experiment with real payment in Ghana. *Malaria Journal, 19*(1), 14. https://doi.org/10.1186/s12936-019-3082-6. Medline:31931828

444 Inungu, J. N., Ankiba, N., Minelli, M., Mumford, V., Bolekela, D., Mukoso, B., Onema, W., Kouton, E., & Raji, D. (2017). Use of insecticide-treated mosquito net among pregnant women and guardians of children under five in the Democratic Republic of the Congo. *Malaria Research and Treatment, 2017*, 5923696. https://doi.org/10.1155/2017/5923696. Medline:29234551

445 Pettifor, A., Taylor, E., Nku, D., Duvall, S., Tabala, M., Meshnick, S., & Behets, F. (2008). Bed net ownership, use and perceptions among women seeking antenatal care in Kinshasa, Democratic Republic of the Congo (DRC): Opportunities for improved maternal and child health. *BMC Public Health, 8*, 331. https://doi.org/10.1186/1471-2458-8-331. Medline:18816373

446 Brooks, H. M., Jean Paul, M. K., Claude, K. M., Mocanu, V., & Hawkes, M. T. (2017). Use and disuse of malaria bed nets in an internally displaced persons camp in the Democratic Republic of the Congo: A mixed-methods study. *PLoS ONE, 12*(9), e0185290. https://doi.org/10.1371/journal.pone.0185290. Medline:28950001

447 World Health Organization. (2013, February 9). *Guidelines for laboratory and field testing of long-lasting insecticidal nets*. https://www.who.int/publications-detail-redirect/9789241505277

448 Ezezika, O., El-Bakri, Y., Nadarajah, A., & Barrett, K. (2022). Implementation of insecticide-treated malaria bed nets in Tanzania: A systematic review. *Journal of Global Health Reports, 6*, e2022036. https://doi.org/10.29392/001c.37363

449 Mathanga, D. P., & Bowie, C. (2007). Malaria control in Malawi: Are the poor being served? *International Journal for Equity in Health, 6*, 22. https://doi.org/10.1186/1475-9276-6-22. Medline:18053158

450 Matovu, F., Goodman, C., Wiseman, V., & Mwengee, W. (2009). How equitable is bed net ownership and utilisation in Tanzania? A practical application of the principles of horizontal and vertical equity. *Malaria Journal, 8*, 109. https://doi.org/10.1186/1475-2875-8-109. Medline:19460153

451 Wacira, D. G., Hill, J., McCall, P. J., & Kroeger, A. (2007). Delivery of insecticide-treated net services through employer and community-based approaches in Kenya. *Tropical Medicine & International Health: TM & IH, 12*(1), 140–149. https://doi.org/10.1111/j.1365-3156.2006.01759.x. Medline:17207158

452 Guyatt, H. L., Ochola, S. A., & Snow, R. W. (2002). Too poor to pay: Charging for insecticide-treated bednets in highland Kenya. *Tropical Medicine & International Health: TM & IH, 7*(10), 846–850. https://doi.org/10.1046/j.1365-3156.2002.00929.x. Medline:12358619

453 Noor, A., Macharia, P., Ouma, P., Oloo, S., Maina, J., Kyalo, D., Olweny, L., Kabaria, C., Kinyoki, D., Snow, R., Erondu, N., Schellenberg, D., Kiptui, R., Njagi, K., Wamari, A., Mbuli, C., Omar, A., & Ejersa, W. (2016). The epidemiology and control profile of malaria in Kenya: Reviewing the evidence to guide the future vector control. https://doi.org/10.13140/RG.2.2.32068.12167

454 Masaninga, F., Mukumbuta, N., Ndhlovu, K., Hamainza, B., Wamulume, P., Chanda, E., Banda, J., Mwanza-Ingwe, M., Miller, J. M., Ameneshewa, B., Mnzava, A., & Kawesha-Chizema, E. (2018). Insecticide-treated nets mass distribution campaign: Benefits and lessons in Zambia. *Malaria Journal, 17*(1), 173. https://doi.org/10.1186/s12936-018-2314-5. Medline:29690873

455 Gingrich, C. D., Hanson, K., Marchant, T., Mulligan, J.-A., & Mponda, H. (2011). Price subsidies and the market for mosquito nets in developing countries: A study of Tanzania's discount voucher scheme. *Social Science & Medicine (1982), 73*(1), 160–168. https://doi.org/10.1016/j.socscimed.2011.04.028. Medline:21684054

456 Magesa, S. M., Lengeler, C., deSavigny, D., Miller, J. E., Njau, R. J., Kramer, K., Kitua, A., & Mwita, A. (2005). Creating an "enabling environment" for taking insecticide treated nets to national scale: The Tanzanian experience. *Malaria Journal, 4*(1), 34. https://doi.org/10.1186/1475-2875-4-34. Medline:16042780

457 Kweku, M., Webster, J., Taylor, I., Burns, S., & Dedzo, M. (2007). Public-private delivery of insecticide-treated nets: A voucher scheme in Volta Region, Ghana. *Malaria Journal, 6*, 14. https://doi.org/10.1186/1475-2875-6-14. Medline:17274810

458 Webster, J., Kweku, M., Dedzo, M., Tinkorang, K., Bruce, J., Lines, J., Chandramohan, D., & Hanson, K. (2010). Evaluating delivery systems: Complex evaluations and plausibility inference. *American Journal of Tropical Medicine and Hygiene, 82*(4), 672–677. https://doi.org/10.4269/ajtmh.2010.09-0473. Medline:20348517

459 Krezanoski, P. J., Comfort, A. B., & Hamer, D. H. (2010). Effect of incentives on insecticide-treated bed net use in sub-Saharan Africa: A

cluster randomized trial in Madagascar. *Malaria Journal, 9*, 186. https://doi.org/10.1186/1475-2875-9-186. Medline:20579392

460 Ricotta, E., Koenker, H., Kilian, A., & Lynch, M. (2014). Are pregnant women prioritized for bed nets? An assessment using survey data from 10 African countries. *Global Health, Science and Practice*, 2(2), 165–172. https://doi.org/10.9745/GHSP-D-14-00021. Medline:25276574

461 Larson, P. S., Eisenberg, J. N. S., Berrocal, V. J., Mathanga, D. P., & Wilson, M. L. (2021). An urban-to-rural continuum of malaria risk: New analytic approaches characterize patterns in Malawi. *Malaria Journal, 20*(1), 418. https://doi.org/10.1186/s12936-021-03950-5. Medline:34689786

462 Hay, S. I., Guerra, C. A., Tatem, A. J., Atkinson, P. M., & Snow, R. W. (2005). Urbanization, malaria transmission and disease burden in Africa. *Nature Reviews. Microbiology, 3*(1), 81–90. https://doi.org/10.1038/nrmicro1069. Medline:15608702

463 Robert, V., Macintyre, K., Keating, J., Trape, J.-F., Duchemin, J.-B., Warren, M., & Beier, J. C. (2003). Malaria transmission in urban Sub-Saharan Africa. *American Journal of Tropical Medicine and Hygiene, 68*(2), 169–176. Medline:12641407

464 Maghendji-Nzondo, S., Kouna, L.-C., Mourembou, G., Boundenga, L., Imboumy-Limoukou, R.-K., Matsiegui, P.-B., Manego-Zoleko, R., Mbatchi, B., Raoult, D., Toure-Ndouo, F., & Lekana-Douki, J. B. (2016). Malaria in urban, semi-urban and rural areas of southern of Gabon: Comparison of the Pfmdr 1 and Pfcrt genotypes from symptomatic children. *Malaria Journal, 15*(1), 420. https://doi.org/10.1186/s12936-016-1469-1. Medline:27538948

465 Molina Gómez, K., Caicedo, M. A., Gaitán, A., Herrera-Varela, M., Arce, M. I., Vallejo, A. F., Padilla, J., Chaparro, P., Pacheco, M. A., Escalante, A. A., Arevalo-Herrera, M., & Herrera, S. (2017). Characterizing the malaria rural-to-urban transmission interface: The importance of reactive case detection. *PLoS Neglected Tropical Diseases, 11*(7), e0005780. https://doi.org/10.1371/journal.pntd.0005780. Medline:28715415

466 Sexton, A. R. (2011). Best practices for an insecticide-treated bed net distribution programme in sub-Saharan eastern Africa. *Malaria Journal, 10*, 157. https://doi.org/10.1186/1475-2875-10-157. Medline:21651815

467 Stanton, M. C., Bockarie, M. J., & Kelly-Hope, L. A. (2013). Geographical factors affecting bed net ownership, a tool for the elimination of Anopheles-transmitted lymphatic filariasis in hard-to-reach communities. *PloS One, 8*(1), e53755. https://doi.org/10.1371/journal.pone.0053755. Medline:23308281

468 Gikandi, P. W., Noor, A. M., Gitonga, C. W., Ajanga, A. A., & Snow, R. W. (2008). Access and barriers to measures targeted to prevent malaria in pregnancy in rural Kenya. *Tropical Medicine & International Health,*

13(2), 208–217. https://doi.org/10.1111/j.1365-3156.2007.01992.x. Medline:18304267

469 Chuma, J., Okungu, V., Ntwiga, J., & Molyneux, C. (2010). Towards achieving Abuja targets: Identifying and addressing barriers to access and use of insecticides treated nets among the poorest populations in Kenya. *BMC Public Health, 10*, 137. https://doi.org/10.1186/1471-2458-10-137. Medline:20233413

470 Onwujekwe, O., Uzochukwu, B., Ezumah, N., & Shu, E. (2005). Increasing coverage of insecticide-treated nets in rural Nigeria: Implications of consumer knowledge, preferences and expenditures for malaria prevention. *Malaria Journal, 4*, 29. https://doi.org/10.1186/1475-2875-4-29. Medline:16026623

471 Eisele, T. P., Thwing, J., & Keating, J. (2011). Claims about the misuse of insecticide-treated mosquito nets: Are these evidence-based? *PLoS Medicine, 8*(4), e1001019. https://doi.org/10.1371/journal.pmed.1001019. Medline:21532734

472 Amoran, O. E., Fatugase, K. O., Fatugase, O. M., & Alausa, K. O. (2012). Impact of health education intervention on insecticide treated nets uptake among nursing mothers in rural communities in Nigeria. *BMC Research Notes, 5*, 444. https://doi.org/10.1186/1756-0500-5-444. Medline:22901329

473 Ndjinga, J. K., & Minakawa, N. (2010). The importance of education to increase the use of bed nets in villages outside of Kinshasa, Democratic Republic of the Congo. *Malaria Journal, 9*, 279. https://doi.org/10.1186/1475-2875-9-279. Medline:20937157

474 U.S. President's Malaria Initiative. (2020, February 4). *Taking malaria education on the road in Ethiopia*. PMI. https://www.pmi.gov/taking-malaria-education-on-the-road-in-ethiopia/

475 Republic of Zambia Ministry of Health. (2011). *National malaria control programme strategic plan for FY 2011–2015 – Consolidating malaria gains for impact*. https://extranet.who.int/countryplanningcycles/sites/default/files/planning_cycle_repository/zambia/zambia_malaria_nsp_2011-2015_.pdf

476 Tweedie, N. (2013, January 18). Bill Gates interview: I have no use for money. This is God's work. *The Telegraph*. https://www.telegraph.co.uk/technology/bill-gates/9812672/Bill-Gates-interview-I-have-no-use-for-money.-This-is-Gods-work.html

477 World Health Organization. (n.d.). *History of polio vaccination*. https://www.who.int/news-room/spotlight/history-of-vaccination/history-of-polio-vaccination

478 Centers for Disease Control and Prevention. (2022, August 3). *Polio elimination in the United States*. https://www.cdc.gov/polio/what-is-polio/polio-us.html

479 Centers for Disease Control and Prevention. (2022, November 3). *Polio vaccination: What everyone should know.* https://www.cdc.gov/vaccines/vpd/polio/public/index.html

480 Centers for Disease Control and Prevention. (2022, December 5). *Polio.* https://www.cdc.gov/polio/vaccines/index.html

481 Pearce, J. M. S. (2004). Salk and Sabin: Poliomyelitis immunisation. *Journal of Neurology, Neurosurgery & Psychiatry, 75*(11), 1552–1552. https://doi.org/10.1136/jnnp.2003.028530

482 Baicus, A. (2012). History of polio vaccination. *World Journal of Virology, 1*(4), 108–114. https://doi.org/10.5501/wjv.v1.i4.108

483 Africa Centers for Disease Control and Prevention. (n.d.). *Poliomyelitis (polio).* https://africacdc.org/disease/poliomyelitis-polio/

484 Wade, M., & Southey, N. (2013). The Poliomyelitis epidemic in Johannesburg in 1918: Medical and public responses. *African Historical Review, 45*(2), 80–112. https://doi.org/10.1080/17532523.2013.857093

485 Poliomyelitis Research Foundation. (n.d.). *How did the Foundation begin | Poliomyelitis Research Foundation.* https://prf.ac.za/home/who-we-are/how-did-the-foundation-begin/

486 World Health Organization. (1997). *Kick polio out of Africa!* https://apps.who.int/iris/bitstream/handle/10665/330798/WH-1997-Nov-Dec-p15-eng.pdf

487 World Health Organization. (n.d.). History of polio vaccination. https://www.who.int/news-room/spotlight/history-of-vaccination/history-of-polio-vaccination

488 Carlisle, D. (1997). National immunisation day. *Africa Health, 20*(1), 10–11. Medline:12348370

489 Africa Kicks Out Wild Polio. (n.d.). *Timeline: Polio eradication in the African region.* https://www.africakicksoutwildpolio.com/timeline/

490 Global Polio Eradication Initiative. (n.d.). *Polio endgame strategy.* https://polioeradication.org/who-we-are/polio-endgame-strategy-2019-2023/

491 Global Polio Eradication Initiative. (2015, September 20). *GPEI – Global eradication of wild poliovirus type 2 declared.* https://polioeradication.org/news-post/global-eradication-of-wild-poliovirus-type-2-declared/

492 UNICEF. (2017, March 24). *From coast to coast: Africa unites to tackle threat of polio.* https://www.unicef.org/press-releases/coast-coast-africa-unites-tackle-threat-polio

493 Mohammed, A., Tomori, O., & Nkengasong, J. N. (2021). Lessons from the elimination of poliomyelitis in Africa. *Nature Reviews. Immunology, 21*(12), 823–828. https://doi.org/10.1038/s41577-021-00640-w. Medline:34697501

494 Global Polio Eradication Initiative. (n.d.). *GPEI – Our mission.* https://polioeradication.org/who-we-are/our-mission/

495 Global Polio Eradication Initiative. (n.d.). *GPEI – Who we are.* https://polioeradication.org/who-we-are/

496 Centers for Disease Control and Prevention. (2022, October 19). *Global Polio Eradication Initiative information.* https://www.cdc.gov/polio/gpei/index.htm

497 World Health Organization Africa. (n.d.). *Polio.* https://www.afro.who.int/health-topics/polio

498 Diop, O. M., Kew, O. M., de Gourville, E. M., & Pallansch, M. A. (2017). The Global Polio Laboratory Network as a platform for the viral vaccine-preventable and emerging Diseases Laboratory Networks. *Journal of Infectious Diseases, 216*(Suppl. 1), S299–S307. https://doi.org/10.1093/infdis/jix092. Medline:28838192

499 Global Polio Eradication Initiative. (n.d.). *GPEI – The Global Polio Laboratory Network.* https://polioeradication.org/polio-today/polio-now/surveillance-indicators/the-global-polio-laboratory-network-gpln/

500 Deressa, W., Kayembe, P., Neel, A. H., Mafuta, E., Seme, A., & Alonge, O. (2020). Lessons learned from the polio eradication initiative in the Democratic Republic of Congo and Ethiopia: Analysis of implementation barriers and strategies. *BMC Public Health, 20*(4), 1807. https://doi.org/10.1186/s12889-020-09879-9. Medline:33339529

501 Nasir, U. N., Bandyopadhyay, A. S., Montagnani, F., Akite, J. E., Mungu, E. B., Uche, I. V., & Ismaila, A. M. (2015). Polio elimination in Nigeria: A review. *Human Vaccines & Immunotherapeutics, 12*(3), 658–663. https://doi.org/10.1080/21645515.2015.1088617. Medline:26383769

502 World Health Organization. (2017). *Report of the 23rd informal consultation of the Global Polio Laboratory Network (GPLN).* https://polioeradication.org/wp-content/uploads/2017/08/GPLN_Meeting_recommendations_2017.pdf

503 Andersen, A., Fisker, A. B., Nielsen, S., Rodrigues, A., Benn, C. S., & Aaby, P. (2021). National immunization campaigns with oral polio vaccine may reduce all-cause mortality: An analysis of 13 years of demographic surveillance data from an urban African area. *Clinical Infectious Diseases: An Official Publication of the Infectious Diseases Society of America, 72*(10), e596–e603. https://doi.org/10.1093/cid/ciaa1351. Medline:32949460

504 World Health Organization. (n.d.). *Poliomyelitis (polio).* https://www.who.int/health-topics/poliomyelitis#tab=tab_1

505 Global Polio Eradication Initiative. (2021). *2020 annual report.* https://polioeradication.org/wp-content/uploads/2021/08/GPEI-2020-Annual-Report-ISBN-9789240030763.pdf

506 Bisrat, F., Kidanel, L., Abraha, K., Asres, M., Dinku, B., Conlon, F., & Fantahun, M. (2013). Cross-border wild polio virus transmission in CORE Group Polio Project areas in Ethiopia. *Ethiopian Medical Journal, 51*(Suppl. 1), 31–39. Medline:24380205

507 Khan, M. U., Ahmad, A., Aqeel, T., Salman, S., Ibrahim, Q., Idrees, J., & Khan, M. U. (2015). Knowledge, attitudes and perceptions towards polio immunization among residents of two highly affected regions of Pakistan. *BMC Public Health, 15*, 1100. https://doi.org/10.1186/s12889-015-2471-1. Medline:26541976

508 Muñoz, D. C., Llamas, L. M., & Bosch-Capblanch, X. (2015). Exposing concerns about vaccination in low- and middle-income countries: A systematic review. *International Journal of Public Health, 60*(7), 767–780. https://doi.org/10.1007/s00038-015-0715-6. Medline:26298444

509 Bedford, J., Chitnis, K., Webber, N., Dixon, P., Limwame, K., Elessawi, R., & Obregon, R. (2017). Community engagement in Liberia: Routine immunization post-Ebola. *Journal of Health Communication, 22*(Suppl. 1), 81–90. https://doi.org/10.1080/10810730.2016.1253122. Medline:28854140

510 Wesseh, C. S., Najjemba, R., Edwards, J. K., Owiti, P., Tweya, H., & Bhat, P. (2017). Did the Ebola outbreak disrupt immunisation services? A case study from Liberia. *Public Health Action, 7*(Suppl. 1), S82–S87. https://doi.org/10.5588/pha.16.0104. Medline:28744444

511 Closser, S., Rosenthal, A., Maes, K., Justice, J., Cox, K., Omidian, P. A., Mohammed, I. Z., Dukku, A. M., Koon, A. D., & Nyirazinyoye, L. (2016). The global context of vaccine refusal: Insights from a systematic comparative ethnography of the Global Polio Eradication initiative. *Medical Anthropology Quarterly, 30*(3), 321–341. https://doi.org/10.1111/maq.12254. Medline:26818631

512 Nuwaha, F., Mulindwa, G., Kabwongyera, E., & Barenzi, J. (2000). Causes of low attendance at national immunization days for polio eradication in Bushenyi district, Uganda. *Tropical Medicine & International Health: TM & IH, 5*(5), 364–369. https://doi.org/10.1046/j.1365-3156.2000.00560.x. Medline:10886801

513 Ezezika, O., Mengistu, M., Opoku, E., Farheen, A., Chauhan, A., & Barrett, K. (2022). What are the barriers and facilitators to polio vaccination and eradication programs? A systematic review. *PLOS Global Public Health, 2*(11), e0001283. https://doi.org/10.1371/journal.pgph.0001283. Medline:36962654

514 Murele, B., Vaz, R., Gasasira, A., Mkanda, P., Erbeto, T., & Okeibunor, J. (2014). Vaccine perception among acceptors and non-acceptors in Sokoto State, Nigeria. *Vaccine, 32*(26), 3323–3327. https://doi.org/10.1016/j.vaccine.2014.03.050. Medline:24713368

515 Ndiaye, S. M., Quick, L., Sanda, O., & Niandou, S. (2003). The value of community participation in disease surveillance: A case study from Niger. *Health Promotion International, 18*(2), 89–98. https://doi.org/10.1093/heapro/18.2.89. Medline:12746380

516 Bangura, J. B., Xiao, S., Qiu, D., Ouyang, F., & Chen, L. (2020). Barriers to childhood immunization in sub-Saharan Africa: A systematic review. *BMC Public Health, 20*(1), 1108. https://doi.org/10.1186/s12889-020-09169-4. Medline:32664849

517 Oku, A., Oyo-Ita, A., Glenton, C., Fretheim, A., Eteng, G., Ames, H., Muloliwa, A., Kaufman, J., Hill, S., Cliff, J., Cartier, Y., Bosch-Capblanch, X., Rada, G., & Lewin, S. (2017). Factors affecting the implementation of childhood vaccination communication strategies in Nigeria: A qualitative study. *BMC Public Health, 17*(1), 200. https://doi.org/10.1186/s12889-017-4020-6. Medline:28202001

518 World Health Organization Africa. (2012). *National immunization days launched*. https://www.afro.who.int/news/national-immunization-days-launched

519 Losey, L., Ogden, E., Bisrat, F., Solomon, R., Newberry, D., Coates, E., Ward, D., Hilmi, L., LeBan, K., Burrowes, V., & Perry, H. B. (2019). The CORE Group Polio Project: An overview of its history and its contributions to the Global Polio Eradication Initiative. *American Journal of Tropical Medicine and Hygiene, 101*(4 Suppl.), 4–14. https://doi.org/10.4269/ajtmh.18-0916. Medline:31760971

520 Utazi, C. E., Thorley, J., Alegana, V. A., Ferrari, M. J., Takahashi, S., Metcalf, C. J. E., Lessler, J., Cutts, F. T., & Tatem, A. J. (2019). Mapping vaccination coverage to explore the effects of delivery mechanisms and inform vaccination strategies. *Nature Communications, 10*(1), 1633. https://doi.org/10.1038/s41467-019-09611-1. Medline:30967543

521 Closser, S., Cox, K., Parris, T. M., Landis, R. M., Justice, J., Gopinath, R., Maes, K., Banteyerga Amaha, H., Mohammed, I. Z., Dukku, A. M., Omidian, P. A., Varley, E., Tedoff, P., Koon, A. D., Nyirazinyoye, L., Luck, M. A., Pont, W. F., Neergheen, V., Rosenthal, A., … Nuttall, E. (2014). The impact of polio eradication on routine immunization and primary health care: A mixed-methods study. *Journal of Infectious Diseases, 210*(Suppl. 1), S504–513. https://doi.org/10.1093/infdis/jit232. Medline:24690667

522 Ghinai, I., Willott, C., Dadari, I., & Larson, H. J. (2013). Listening to the rumours: What the northern Nigeria polio vaccine boycott can tell us ten years on. *Global Public Health, 8*(10), 1138–1150. https://doi.org/10.1080/17441692.2013.859720. Medline:24294986

523 Bozzola, E., Spina, G., Russo, R., Bozzola, M., Corsello, G., & Villani, A. (2018). Mandatory vaccinations in European countries, undocumented information, false news and the impact on vaccination uptake: The position of the Italian pediatric society. *Italian Journal of Pediatrics, 44*(1), 67. https://doi.org/10.1186/s13052-018-0504-y. Medline:29898770

524 Chung, Y., Schamel, J., Fisher, A., & Frew, P. M. (2017). Influences on immunization decision-making among US parents of young children.

Maternal and Child Health Journal, 21(12), 2178–2187. https://doi.org/10.1007/s10995-017-2336-6. Medline:28755045

525 Shen, S. C., & Dubey, V. (2019). Addressing vaccine hesitancy: Clinical guidance for primary care physicians working with parents. *Canadian Family Physician Medecin De Famille Canadien, 65*(3), 175–181. Medline:30867173

526 Onnela, J.-P., Landon, B. E., Kahn, A.-L., Ahmed, D., Verma, H., O'Malley, A. J., Bahl, S., Sutter, R. W., & Christakis, N. A. (2016). Polio vaccine hesitancy in the networks and neighborhoods of Malegaon, India. *Social Science & Medicine (1982), 153*, 99–106. https://doi.org/10.1016/j.socscimed.2016.01.024. Medline:26889952

527 Rosenstein, N. E., Perkins, B. A., Stephens, D. S., Popovic, T., & Hughes, J. M. (2001). Meningococcal disease. *New England Journal of Medicine, 344*(18), 1378–1388. https://doi.org/10.1056/NEJM200105033441807. Medline:28364047

528 Mazamay, S., Guégan, J.-F., Diallo, N., Bompangue, D., Bokabo, E., Muyembe, J.-J., Taty, N., Vita, T. P., & Broutin, H. (2021). An overview of bacterial meningitis epidemics in Africa from 1928 to 2018 with a focus on epidemics "outside-the-belt." *BMC Infectious Diseases, 21*(1), 1027. https://doi.org/10.1186/s12879-021-06724-1. Medline:34592937

529 Soeters, H. M., Diallo, A. O., Bicaba, B. W., Kadadé, G., Dembélé, A. Y., Acyl, M. A., Nikiema, C., Sadji, A. Y., Poy, A. N., Lingani, C., Tall, H., Sakandé, S., Tarbangdo, F., Aké, F., Mbaeyi, S. A., Moïsi, J., Paye, M. F., Sanogo, Y. O., Vuong, J. T., … Novak, R. T. (2019). Bacterial meningitis epidemiology in 5 countries in the Meningitis Belt of sub-Saharan Africa, 2015–2017. *Journal of Infectious Diseases, 220*(Suppl. 4), S165–S174. https://doi.org/10.1093/infdis/jiz358. Medline:31671441

530 Zunt, J. R., Kassebaum, N. J., Blake, N., Glennie, L., Wright, C., Nichols, E., Abd-Allah, F., Abdela, J., Abdelalim, A., Adamu, A. A., Adib, M. G., Ahmadi, A., Ahmed, M. B., Aichour, A. N., Aichour, I., Aichour, M. T. E., Akseer, N., Al-Raddadi, R. M., Alahdab, F., … Murray, C. J. L. (2018). Global, regional, and national burden of meningitis, 1990–2016: A systematic analysis for the Global Burden of Disease Study 2016. *The Lancet Neurology, 17*(12), 1061–1082. https://doi.org/10.1016/S1474-4422(18)30387-9. Medline:30507391

531 Fernandez, K., Lingani, C., Aderinola, O. M., Goumbi, K., Bicaba, B., Edea, Z. A., Glèlè, C., Sarkodie, B., Tamekloe, A., Ngomba, A., Djingarey, M., Bwaka, A., Perea, W., & Ronveaux, O. (2019). Meningococcal meningitis outbreaks in the African Meningitis Belt after meningococcal serogroup A conjugate vaccine introduction, 2011–2017. *Journal of Infectious Diseases, 220*(Suppl. 4), S225–S232. https://doi.org/10.1093/infdis/jiz355. Medline:31671449

532 Mustapha, M. M., & Harrison, L. H. (2018). Vaccine prevention of meningococcal disease in Africa: Major advances, remaining challenges. *Human Vaccines & Immunotherapeutics, 14*(5), 1107–1115. https://doi.org/10.1080/21645515.2017.1412020. Medline:29211624

533 Garba, M., & Abidakun, M. (2021, September 10). *Nigeria: The infamous 1996 Pfizer trial driving anti-vax feelings today*. African Arguments. https://africanarguments.org/2021/09/nigeria-the-infamous-1996-pfizer-trial-driving-anti-vax-feelings-today/

534 Domingo, P., Pomar, V., Mauri, A., & Barquet, N. (2019). Standing on the shoulders of giants: Two centuries of struggle against meningococcal disease. *The Lancet Infectious Diseases, 19*(8), e284–e294. https://doi.org/10.1016/S1473-3099(19)30040-4. Medline:31053493

535 Frederiks, J. A., & Koehler, P. J. (1997). The first lumbar puncture. *Journal of the History of the Neurosciences, 6*(2), 147–153. https://doi.org/10.1080/09647049709525699. Medline:11619518

536 Mandal, A. (2009). *History of meningitis*. News-Medical.Net. https://www.news-medical.net/health/History-of-Meningitis.aspx

537 De Wals, P. (2004). Meningococcal C vaccines: The Canadian experience. *Pediatric Infectious Disease Journal, 23*(12 Suppl.), S280–284. Medline:15597070

538 PATH. (2015). *The meningitis vaccine project: A groundbreaking partnership*. https://www.path.org/articles/about-meningitis-vaccine-project/

539 United Nations. (2022, September 8). *UN health agency kicks off meningitis vaccination campaigns in Africa*. UN News. https://news.un.org/en/story/2022/09/1126231

540 World Health Organization. (2021, September 28). *Meningitis*. https://www.who.int/news-room/fact-sheets/detail/meningitis

541 World Health Organization. (2021, September 20). *Meningitis – Democratic Republic of the Congo*. https://www.who.int/emergencies/disease-outbreak-news/item/2021-DON334

542 World Health Organization. (2022, September 8). *COVID-19 threatens elimination of deadly form of meningitis in Africa, more than 50 million children miss vaccination*. Regional Office for Africa. https://www.afro.who.int/news/covid-19-threatens-elimination-deadly-form-meningitis-africa-more-50-million-children-miss

543 Zeitvogel, K. (2016, June). *MenAfriVac vaccine slashes meningitis cases in Africa*. Fogarty International Center. https://www.fic.nih.gov:443/News/GlobalHealthMatters/may-june-2016/Pages/menafrivac-meningitis-vaccine.aspx

544 Jaca, A., Wiyeh, A. B., Sambala, E. Z., & Wiysonge, C. S. (2021). The burden of meningococcal meningitis in the African Meningitis Belt, from 2009 to 2014: A trend analysis. *Pan African Medical Journal, 39*, 57. https://doi.org/10.11604/pamj.2021.39.57.17629. Medline:34422180

545 Trotter, C. L., Lingani, C., Fernandez, K., Cooper, L. V., Bita, A., Tevi-Benissan, C., Ronveaux, O., Préziosi, M.-P., & Stuart, J. M. (2017). Impact of MenAfriVac in nine countries of the African Meningitis Belt, 2010–15: An analysis of surveillance data. *The Lancet Infectious Diseases, 17*(8), 867–872. https://doi.org/10.1016/S1473-3099(17)30301-8. Medline:28545721

546 Viviani, S. (2022). Efficacy and effectiveness of the meningococcal conjugate group A vaccine MenAfriVac® in preventing recurrent meningitis epidemics in Sub-Saharan Africa. *Vaccines, 10*(4), Article 4. https://doi.org/10.3390/vaccines10040617. Medline:35455366

547 Ezezika, O., Mengistu, M., & Lear, T. (2021). Implementation of the Meningitis Vaccine Project in Africa: Lessons for vaccine implementation programs. *Journal of Global Health Reports, 5*, e2021097. https://doi.org/10.29392/001c.29042

548 Cunningham, M. S., Davison, C., & Aronson, K. J. (2014). HPV vaccine acceptability in Africa: A systematic review. *Preventive Medicine, 69*, 274–279. https://doi.org/10.1016/j.ypmed.2014.08.035. Medline:25451327

549 Amponsah-Dacosta, E., Blose, N., Nkwinika, V. V., & Chepkurui, V. (2022). Human papillomavirus vaccination in South Africa: Programmatic challenges and opportunities for integration with other adolescent health services? *Frontiers in Public Health, 10*, 799984. https://doi.org/10.3389/fpubh.2022.799984. Medline:35174123

550 GAVI. (n.d.). *Rwanda*. Retrieved November 18, 2022, from https://www.gavi.org/programmes-impact/country-hub/africa/rwanda

551 GAVI. (2022). *Human papillomavirus*. https://www.gavi.org/types-support/vaccine-support/human-papillomavirus

552 Forman, D., de Martel, C., Lacey, C. J., Soerjomataram, I., Lortet-Tieulent, J., Bruni, L., Vignat, J., Ferlay, J., Bray, F., Plummer, M., & Franceschi, S. (2012). Global burden of human papillomavirus and related diseases. *Vaccine, 30*(Suppl. 5), F12–23. https://doi.org/10.1016/j.vaccine.2012.07.055. Medline:23199955

553 Kombe Kombe, A. J., Li, B., Zahid, A., Mengist, H. M., Bounda, G.-A., Zhou, Y., & Jin, T. (2021). Epidemiology and burden of human papillomavirus and related diseases, molecular pathogenesis, and vaccine evaluation. *Frontiers in Public Health, 8*, 552028. https://doi.org/10.3389/fpubh.2020.552028. Medline:33553082

554 Bruni, L., Albero, G., Serrano, B., Mena, M., Collado, J. J., Gomez, D., Munoz, J., Bosch, F. X., & de Sanjose, S. (2021). *Human papillomavirus and related diseases report*. ICO/IARC Information Centre on HPV and Cancer (HPV Information Centre). https://hpvcentre.net/statistics/reports/XFX.pdf?t=1569498678112

555 Sung, H., Ferlay, J., Siegel, R. L., Laversanne, M., Soerjomataram, I., Jemal, A., & Bray, F. (2021). Global cancer statistics 2020: GLOBOCAN

estimates of incidence and mortality worldwide for 36 cancers in 185 countries. *CA: A Cancer Journal for Clinicians, 71*(3), 209–249. https://doi.org/10.3322/caac.21660. Medline:33538338

556 Missaoui, N., Trabelsi, A., Parkin, D. M., Jaidene, L., Chatti, D., Mokni, M., Korbi, S., & Hmissa, S. (2010). Trends in the incidence of cancer in the Sousse region, Tunisia, 1993–2006. *International Journal of Cancer, 127*(11), 2669–2677. https://doi.org/10.1002/ijc.25490. Medline:20521249

557 Union for International Cancer Control. (2022). *Cervical cancer elimination in Africa: Where are we now and where do.* https://www.uicc.org/news/cervical-cancer-elimination-africa-where-are-we-now-and-where-do-we-need-be

558 Jedy-Agba, E., Joko, W. Y., Liu, B., Buziba, N. G., Borok, M., Korir, A., Masamba, L., Manraj, S. S., Finesse, A., Wabinga, H., Somdyala, N., & Parkin, D. M. (2020). Trends in cervical cancer incidence in sub-Saharan Africa. *British Journal of Cancer, 123*(1), Article 1. https://doi.org/10.1038/s41416-020-0831-9. Medline:32336751

559 Vaccarella, S., Laversanne, M., Ferlay, J., & Bray, F. (2017). Cervical cancer in Africa, Latin America and the Caribbean and Asia: Regional inequalities and changing trends. *International Journal of Cancer, 141*(10), 1997–2001. https://doi.org/10.1002/ijc.30901. Medline:28734013

560 Montefiore Medical Center. (2022). *Long-term human papillomavirus vaccination effectiveness and immunity in Rwandan women living with and without human immunodeficiency virus* (Clinical Trial Registration No. NCT05247853). clinicaltrials.gov. https://clinicaltrials.gov/ct2/show/NCT05247853

561 Delany-Moretlwe, S., Kelley, K. F., James, S., Scorgie, F., Subedar, H., Dlamini, N. R., Pillay, Y., Naidoo, N., Chikandiwa, A., & Rees, H. (2018). Human Papillomavirus vaccine introduction in South Africa: Implementation lessons from an evaluation of the national school-based vaccination campaign. *Global Health: Science and Practice, 6*(3), 425–438. https://doi.org/10.9745/GHSP-D-18-00090. Medline:30143561

562 Tan, N., Sharma, M., Winer, R., Galloway, D., Rees, H., & Barnabas, R. V. (2018). Model-estimated effectiveness of single dose 9-valent HPV vaccination for HIV-positive and HIV-negative females in South Africa. *Vaccine, 36*(32 Pt A), 4830–4836. https://doi.org/10.1016/j.vaccine.2018.02.023. Medline:29891348

563 World Health Organization. (2022, November 17). *Cervical cancer elimination initiative.* https://www.who.int/initiatives/cervical-cancer-elimination-initiative

564 Barnabas, R. V., Brown, E. R., Onono, M. A., Bukusi, E. A., Njoroge, B., Winer, R. L., Galloway, D. A., Pinder, L. F., Donnell, D., Wakhungu, I., Congo, O., Biwott, C., Kimanthi, S., Oluoch, L., Heller, K. B., Leingang,

H., Morrison, S., Rechkina, E., Cherne, S., … Mugo, N. (2022). Efficacy of single-dose HPV vaccination among young African women. *NEJM Evidence, 1*(5), EVIDoa2100056. https://doi.org/10.1056/EVIDoa2100056. Medline:35693874

565 Lei, J., Ploner, A., Elfström, K. M., Wang, J., Roth, A., Fang, F., Sundström, K., Dillner, J., & Sparén, P. (2020). HPV vaccination and the risk of invasive cervical cancer. *New England Journal of Medicine, 383*(14), 1340–1348. https://doi.org/10.1056/NEJMoa1917338. Medline:32997908

566 Palmer, T., Wallace, L., Pollock, K. G., Cuschieri, K., Robertson, C., Kavanagh, K., & Cruickshank, M. (2019). Prevalence of cervical disease at age 20 after immunisation with bivalent HPV vaccine at age 12–13 in Scotland: Retrospective population study. *BMJ, 365*, l1161. https://doi.org/10.1136/bmj.l1161. Medline:30944092

567 Dereje, N., Gebremariam, A., Addissie, A., Worku, A., Assefa, M., Abraha, A., Tigeneh, W., Kantelhardt, E. J., & Jemal, A. (2020). Factors associated with advanced stage at diagnosis of cervical cancer in Addis Ababa, Ethiopia: A population-based study. *BMJ Open, 10*(10), e040645. https://doi.org/10.1136/bmjopen-2020-040645. Medline:33051237

568 Ibrahim, A., Rasch, V., Pukkala, E., & Aro, A. R. (2011). Predictors of cervical cancer being at an advanced stage at diagnosis in Sudan. *International Journal of Women's Health, 3*, 385–389. https://doi.org/10.2147/IJWH.S21063. Medline:22140326

569 Seraphin, T. P., Joko-Fru, W. Y., Manraj, S. S., Chokunonga, E., Somdyala, N. I. M., Korir, A., N'Da, G., Finesse, A., Wabinga, H., Assefa, M., Gnangnon, F., Hansen, R., Buziba, N. G., Liu, B., Kantelhardt, E. J., & Parkin, D. M. (2021). Prostate cancer survival in sub-Saharan Africa by age, stage at diagnosis, and human development index: A population-based registry study. *Cancer Causes & Control: CCC, 32*(9), 1001–1019. https://doi.org/10.1007/s10552-021-01453-x. Medline:34244896

570 McClung, N., Mathoma, A., Gargano, J. W., Nyepetsi, N. G., Querec, T. D., Onyekwuluje, J., Mine, M., Morroni, C., Luckett, R., Markowitz, L. E., & Ramogola-Masire, D. (2022). HPV prevalence among young adult women living with and without HIV in Botswana for future HPV vaccine impact monitoring. *BMC Infectious Diseases, 22*(1), 176. https://doi.org/10.1186/s12879-022-07130-x. Medline:35193517

571 Liu, G., Mugo, N. R., Bayer, C., Rao, D. W., Onono, M., Mgodi, N. M., Chirenje, Z. M., Njoroge, B. W., Tan, N., Bukusi, E. A., & Barnabas, R. V. (2022). Impact of catch-up human papillomavirus vaccination on cervical cancer incidence in Kenya: A mathematical modeling evaluation of HPV vaccination strategies in the context of moderate HIV prevalence. *EClinicalMedicine, 45*. https://doi.org/10.1016/j.eclinm.2022.101306. Medline:35243272

572 Abbas, K. M., van Zandvoort, K., Brisson, M., & Jit, M. (2020). Effects of updated demography, disability weights, and cervical cancer burden on estimates of human papillomavirus vaccination impact at the global, regional, and national levels: A PRIME modelling study. *The Lancet Global Health*, *8*(4), e536–e544. https://doi.org/10.1016/S2214-109X(20)30022-X. Medline:32105613

573 Sayinzoga, F., Tenet, V., Heideman, D. A. M., Sibomana, H., Umulisa, M.-C., Franceschi, S., Hakizimana, J. de D., Clifford, G. M., & Baussano, I. (2023). Human papillomavirus vaccine effect against human papillomavirus infection in Rwanda: Evidence from repeated cross-sectional cervical-cell-based surveys. *The Lancet Global Health*, *11*(7), e1096–e1104. https://doi.org/10.1016/S2214-109X(23)00193-6

574 Murenzi, G., & Mungo, C. (2023). Impact of the human papillomavirus vaccine in low-resource settings. *The Lancet. Global Health*, *11*(7), e997–e998. https://doi.org/10.1016/S2214-109X(23)00203-6

575 MERCK. (2013). *GARDASIL® [human papillomavirus quadrivalent (Types 6, 11, 16, and 18) Vaccine, Recombinant], Merck's HPV vaccine, available to developing countries through UNICEF Tender*. Merck.Com. https://www.merck.com/news/gardasil-human-papillomavirus-quadrivalent-types-6-11-16-and-18-vaccine-recombinant-mercks-hpv-vaccine-available-to-developing-countries-through-unicef-tender/

576 Ezezika, O., Purwaha, M., Patel, H., & Mengistu, M. (2022). The human papillomavirus vaccine project in Rwanda: Lessons for vaccine implementation effectiveness. *Global Implementation Research and Applications*, 2, 394–403.

577 Binagwaho, A., Wagner, C. M., Gatera, M., Karema, C., Nutt, C. T., & Ngabo, F. (2012). Achieving high coverage in Rwanda's national human papillomavirus vaccination programme. *Bulletin of the World Health Organization*, *90*(8), 623–628. https://doi.org/10.2471/BLT.11.097253. Medline:22893746

578 PATH, CHDC, & UNEPI. (2011). HPV vaccination in Africa: Lessons learned from a pilot program in Uganda. *Seattle: PATH, 28*.

579 Republic of Rwanda Ministry of Education. (2012). *2011 education statistics*. https://businessprocedures.rdb.rw/media/2011_EDUCATION_STATISTICS_Jan_2012.pdf

580 LaMontagne, D. S., Bloem, P. J. N., Brotherton, J. M. L., Gallagher, K. E., Badiane, O., & Ndiaye, C. (n.d.). Progress in HPV vaccination in low- and lower-middle-income countries. *International Journal of Gynecology & Obstetrics*, *138*(S1), 7–14. https://doi.org/10.1002/ijgo.12186. Medline:28691329

581 Cousins, S. (2019). *Why Rwanda could be the first country to wipe out cervical cancer*. CNN. https://www.cnn.com/2019/05/30/health/rwanda-first-eliminate-cervical-cancer-africa-partner

582 Republic of Rwanda Ministry of Health, & WHO Africa. (n.d.). *Rwanda's performance in addressing social determinants of health and intersectoral action*. https://www.afro.who.int/sites/default/files/2018-03/Rwanda_s_Performance_in_Addressing_Social_Determinants_of_Health__and%20intersectoral%20action%20final%20Report.pdf

583 World Health Organization. (2024, October 20). *Africa immunization advisory group urges single-dose HPV vaccine adoption to advance vaccination efforts*. Regional Office for Africa. https://www.afro.who.int/news/africa-immunization-advisory-group-urges-single-dose-hpv-vaccine-adoption-advance-vaccination

584 Karanja-Chege, C. M. (2022). HPV vaccination in Kenya: The challenges faced and strategies to increase uptake. *Frontiers in Public Health, 10*, 802947. https://doi.org/10.3389/fpubh.2022.802947

585 Becker-Dreps, S., Otieno, W. A., Brewer, N. T., Agot, K., & Smith, J. S. (2010). HPV vaccine acceptability among Kenyan women. *Vaccine, 28*(31), 4864. https://doi.org/10.1016/j.vaccine.2010.05.034

586 Watson-Jones, D., Tomlin, K., Remes, P., Baisley, K., Ponsiano, R., Soteli, S., de Sanjosé, S., Changalucha, J., Kapiga, S., & Hayes, R. J. (2012). Reasons for receiving or not receiving HPV vaccination in primary schoolgirls in Tanzania: A case control study. *PloS One*, *7*(10), e45231. https://doi.org/10.1371/journal.pone.0045231

587 Centers for Disease Control and Prevention. (2021, February 21). *History of smallpox*. https://www.cdc.gov/smallpox/history/history.html

588 Fenner, F., Henderson, D. A., Arita, I., Jezek, Z., Ladnyi, I. D., & Organization, W. H. (1988). *Smallpox and its eradication*. World Health Organization. https://apps.who.int/iris/handle/10665/39485

589 Breman, J. G. (2021). Smallpox eradication: African origin, African solutions, and relevance for COVID-19. *American Journal of Tropical Medicine and Hygiene, 104*(2), 416–421. https://doi.org/10.4269/ajtmh.20-1557. Medline:33534731

590 Fenner, F. (1982). A successful eradication campaign: Global eradication of smallpox. *Reviews of Infectious Diseases*, *4*(5), 916–930.

591 Henderson, D. A., & Klepac, P. (2013). Lessons from the eradication of smallpox: An interview with DA Henderson. *Philosophical Transactions of the Royal Society B, 368*(1623), 1–7. https://doi.org/10.1098/rstb.2013.0113. Medline:23798700

592 Henderson, D. A. (2009). *Smallpox: The death of a disease—The inside story of eradicating a worldwide killer*. Prometheus Books.

593 Hinman, A. R. (1998). Global progress in infectious disease control. *Vaccine, 16*(11–12), 1116–1121. https://doi.org/10.1016/S0264-410X(98)80107-2. Medline:9682367

594 Barrett, S. (2013). Economic considerations for the eradication endgame. *Philosophical Transactions of the Royal Society B: Biological*

Sciences, 368(1623), 20120149. https://doi.org/10.1098/rstb.2012.0149. Medline:23798697

595 Barrett, S. (2007). The smallpox eradication game. *Public Choice, 130*(1/2), 179–207. http://www.jstor.org/stable/27698049

596 Merck. (2023, August 3). *U.S.FDA approves Merck's ERVEBO® (Ebola Zaire vaccine, live) for Use in children 12 months of age and older* [Press release]. https://www.merck.com/news/u-s-fda-approves-mercks-ervebo-ebola-zaire-vaccine-live-for-use-in-children-12-months-of-age-and-older/

597 GAVI. (2021, January 12). *500,000 doses of Ebola vaccine to be made available to countries for outbreak response.* https://www.gavi.org/news/media-room/500000-doses-ebola-vaccine-be-made-available-countries-outbreak-response

598 Wells, C. R., Pandey, A., Parpia, A. S., Fitzpatrick, M. C., Meyers, L. A., Singer, B. H., & Galvani, A. P. (2019). Ebola vaccination in the Democratic Republic of the Congo. *Proceedings of the National Academy of Sciences of the United States of America, 116*(20), 10178–10183. https://doi.org/10.1073/pnas.1817329116. Medline:31036657

599 World Health Organization. (2018, December 12). *Ebola virus disease: Democratic Republic of Congo: External situation report 19.* https://www.who.int/publications-detail-redirect/ebola-virus-disease-democratic-republic-of-congo-external-situation-report-19-2018

600 World Health Organization. (2018). *Ebola virus disease: Democratic Republic of Congo. External situation report 14.* https://apps.who.int/iris/bitstream/handle/10665/272997/SITREP_EVD_DRC_20180701-eng.pdf

601 World Health Organization. (2018). *Ebola virus disease: Democratic Republic of Congo: External situation report 17.* https://apps.who.int/iris/bitstream/handle/10665/273348/SITREP_EVD_DRC_20180725-eng.pdf

602 World Health Organization. (2019, May 7). *World Health Organization adapts Ebola vaccination strategy in the Democratic Republic of the Congo to account for insecurity and community feedback.* https://www.who.int/news/item/07-05-2019-who-adapts-ebola-vaccination-strategy-in-the-democratic-republic-of-the-congo-to-account-for-insecurity-and-community-feedback

603 World Health Organization. (2019, April 13). *Preliminary results on the efficacy of rVSV-ZEBOV-GP Ebola vaccine using the ring vaccination strategy in the control of an Ebola outbreak in the Democratic Republic of the Congo: An example of integration of research into epidemic response.* https://reliefweb.int/report/democratic-republic-congo/preliminary-results-efficacy-rvsv-zebov-gp-ebola-vaccine-using-ring

604 World Bank. (2022). *Current health expenditure (% of GDP).* https://data.worldbank.org/indicator/SH.XPD.CHEX.GD.ZS

605 Novignon, J., Olakojo, S. A., & Nonvignon, J. (2012). The effects of public and private health care expenditure on health status in sub-Saharan Africa: New evidence from panel data analysis. *Health Economics Review*, *2*(1), 1–8. https://doi.org/10.1186/2191-1991-2-22/TABLES/6. Medline:23232089

606 Azevedo, M. J. (2017). The State of Health System(s) in Africa: Challenges and Opportunities. In M. J. Azevedo (Ed.), Historical Perspectives on the State of Health and Health Systems in Africa, Volume II: The Modern Era (pp. 1–73). Springer International Publishing. https://doi.org/10.1007/978-3-319-32564-4_1

607 Kirkup, B. (2009). Scaling up health service delivery – From pilot innovations to policies and programmes. *Public Health*, *123*(9), 638–639. https://doi.org/10.1016/j.puhe.2009.05.012

608 World Health Organization. (2021). *Global expenditure on health: Public spending on the rise?* World Health Organization. https://apps.who.int/iris/handle/10665/350560

609 World Bank. (2021). *World Bank's response to COVID-19 (coronavirus) in Africa* https://www.worldbank.org/en/news/factsheet/2020/06/02/world-banks-response-to-covid-19-coronavirus-in-africa

610 World Bank. (2022). *Current health expenditure per capita (current US$) – Sub-Saharan Africa | Data*. https://data.worldbank.org/indicator/SH.XPD.CHEX.PC.CD?locations=ZG

611 Institute for Health Metrics and Evaluation. (2021). *Financing global health.* http://vizhub.healthdata.org/fgh

612 Sarkar, S., Corso, P., Ebrahim-Zadeh, S., Kim, P., Charania, S., & Wall, K. (2019). Cost-effectiveness of HIV prevention interventions in Sub-Saharan Africa: A systematic review. *EClinicalMedicine*, *10*, 10–31. https://doi.org/10.1016/j.eclinm.2019.04.006. Medline:31193863

613 World Bank. (2022). *Current health expenditure per capita (current US$)*. https://data.worldbank.org/indicator/SH.XPD.CHEX.PC.CD

614 UNESCO Institute for Statistics. (n.d.). *UIS Statistics*. Retrieved 22 October 2024, from https://dta.uis.unesco.org/

615 Montgomery, S. (2021). *CIRGO Initiative blazes trail in global health.* https://criticalvalues.org/news/all/2022/09/30/cirgo-initiative-blazes-trail-in-global-health

616 Montgomery, S. (2021, December 20). *Minding the gaps: Implementation science research for improved cancer care in Africa*. https://criticalvalues.org/news/item/2021/12/20/minding-the-gaps-implementation-science-research-for-improved-cancer-care-in-africa

617 Ezezika, O. C. (2015). Building trust: A critical component of global health. *Annals of Global Health*, *81*(5), 589–592. https://doi.org/10.1016/j.aogh.2015.12.007

605 Novignon, J., Olakojo, S. A., & Nonvignon, J. (2012). The effects of public and private health care expenditure on health status in sub-Saharan Africa: New evidence from panel data analysis. *Health Economics Review, 2*(1), 1–8. https://doi.org/10.1186/2191-1991-2-22 Medline:23232089

606 [illegible], M. J. (2017). The state of health systems in Africa: Challenges and Opportunities. In M. J. Azevedo (Ed.), *Historical Perspectives on the State of Health and Health Systems in Africa, Volume II: The Modern Era* (pp. [illegible]). Springer International Publishing. https://doi.org/10.1007/978-3-319-32564-4_[illegible]

607 Kirigia, [illegible] (2009). Scaling up health service delivery – From pilot innovations to policies and programmes. *Public Health, 123*(9), 638–639. https://doi.org/10.1016/j.puhe.2009.05.012

608 World Health Organization. (2021). *Global expenditure on health: Public spending on the rise?* World Health Organization. https://apps.who.int/iris/handle/10665/350560

609 World Bank. (2020). *World Bank's response to COVID-19 (coronavirus) in Africa*. https://www.worldbank.org/en/news/factsheet/2020/06/02/world-banks-response-to-covid-19-coronavirus-in-africa

610 World Bank. (2022). *Current health expenditure per capita (current US$) – Sub-Saharan Africa | Data*. https://data.worldbank.org/indicator/SH.XPD.CHEX.PC.CD?locations=ZG

611 Institute for Health Metrics and Evaluation. (2020). *Financing global health*. http://vizhub.healthdata.org/fgh

612 Barker, S., [illegible], P., Ebrahimi-Zadeh, S., Kim, J., Chaudhury, S., & [illegible], R. (2019). Cost-effectiveness of HIV prevention interventions in Sub-Saharan Africa: A systematic review. *EClinicalMedicine, 10*, 10–31. https://doi.org/10.1016/j.eclinm.2019.04.015 Medline:31193863

613 World Bank. (2022). *[illegible]*. https://data.worldbank.org/indicator/SH.XPD.CHEX.PC.CD

614 UNESCO Institute for Statistics. (n.d.). *UIS Statistics*. Retrieved 22 October 2021, from http://data.uis.unesco.org/

615 [illegible], S. (2022). [illegible] global health. https://[illegible]/news/2022/09/30/[illegible]-in-global-health

616 Montgomery, S. (2021, December 20). *Minding the gaps: Implementation science research for improved cancer care in Africa*. https://[illegible]/news/2021/12/20/minding-the-gaps-implementation-science-research-for-improved-cancer-care-in-africa

617 [illegible], O. S. (2015). Building trust: A critical component of global health. *Annals of Global Health, 81*(5), 589–592. https://doi.org/10.1016/j.aogh.2015.12.007